Take Charge of Your Health!
Self-Assessment Workbook with Review and Practice Tests

for

Donatelle

Access to Health

Seventh Edition

Self-Assessments prepared by
Judy Baker
Chico State University

Practice Tests prepared by
Lynne Blesz Vestal

Benjamin Cummings

San Francisco Boston New York
Capetown Hong Kong London Madrid Mexico City
Montreal Munich Paris Singapore Sydney Tokyo Toronto

ISBN 0-205-34635-9

Benjamin Cummings

12345678910 0605040302

www.aw.com/bc

Table of Contents

Health Improvement Project 1
Health Improvement Contract 2
Health Improvement Evaluation 4
Martin's Index of Health Behavior 5
Life-Orientation Test 10
Multidimensional Health Locus of Control 12
Getting Started: Self-Assessment 14
What Health Screening Examinations Do You Need? 16
Personal Information Form 17
Personal Prevention Record 18
Medication Record 19
Develop Your Own Support System 20
Self-Esteem Inventory-Part I 21
Self-Esteem Inventory-Part II Personal Application 23
Need for Uniqueness Scale 25
Self-Actualization Inventory 27
How Hardy Are You? 29
Inventory of Negative Thoughts 31
Assertiveness Scale 33
Could You Have Panic Disorder? 36
Anxiety Symptoms Checklist 37
Satisfaction with Life Scale 38
People in Your Life 39
Assessing and Managing Stress 41
A Time Management Questionnaire for College Students 43
How Do You Handle Conflict? 45
Constructive Fighting 49
Test Your Sleep I.Q. 52
The Family Stress Test: How Stressed is Your Family? 55
How You Deal with Your Stress 57
Your Ideas About Decisions 61

Rating the Evening News: Aggressive and Prosocial Acts 63
Coercive Sex Questionnaire 65
Household Poison Safety Checklist 69
Can Your Kitchen Pass the Food Safety Test? 71
Home Safety Checklist 74
Characteristics of Perpetrators of Workplace Violence 81
Does She Have a Safety Plan? 82
Can You Help Survivors of Homicide? 83
Types of Love 85
Are You and Your Partner Suited for a Life Together? 86
Getting to Know Your Own Level of Trust 92
Needs in Close Relationships 94
Muehlenhard-Quackenbush Sexual Attitude Survey 96
Index of Sexual Satisfaction 98
Love and Sex 100
Parent? Inventory 101
Should You Have the HIV Test? 103
Are You Ready for a Healthy Pregnancy? 104
Rating Your Diet 105
Daily Food Diary 111
Your Eating Habits and Extra Calories 112
Why Do You Eat? Inventory 114
Do You Have an Eating Disorder? 117
Check Your Cholesterol and Heart Disease I.Q. 119
Your Exercise Contract 122
How Much Do I Move? 124
Check Your Physical Activity & Heart Disease I.Q. 126
The Muscle Hustle: Test Your Exercise I.Q. 129
Marijuana Attitudes 131
Why People Use Drugs 132
Do You Have a Drug Problem? 133
Evaluating Drug Use Presentation in Movies 135
Passive Smoking 137
Is Someone You Know an Inhalant Abuser? 138

Drinking Related Internal-External Locus of Control Scale 139
The CAGE Questionnaire 143
Alcohol Effects Questionnaire 144
Why Do You Smoke? 147
Beliefs About Smoking 149
Check Your High Blood Pressure Prevention IQ 151
Check Your Healthy Heart I.Q. 154
Your Risk of STDs 158
Check Your Asthma I.Q. 160
Check Your Blood I.Q. 163
Chronic Fatigue Syndrome Symptoms Checklist 165
How Accurate Are Your Perceptions of Aging? 166
I'd Pick More Daisies 168
Ten Ways To Recognize Hearing Loss 169
Take This Eye-Q Test 170
Death and Life's Human Relationships 172
Environmental Quiz 174
Checklist for the Prevention of Carbon Monoxide (CO) Poisoning 178
Checkup on Health Insurance Choices: Which Type Is Right for You? 180
Choosing a Doctor 181
Making Decisions about Surgery 185
Choosing a Health Plan 186
Choosing Treatments 189

Review and Practice Tests

Chapter 1 Promoting Healthy Behavior Change A-1
Chapter 2 Psychosocial Health A-4
Chapter 3 Managing Stress A-7
Chapter 4 Violence and Abuse A-10
Chapter 5 Healthy Relationships A-13
Chapter 6 Sexuality A-16
Chapter 7 Reproductive Choices A-19
Chapter 8 Nutrition A-22
Chapter 9 Managing Your Weight A-25

Chapter 10 Personal Fitness A-28

Chapter 11 Addictions and Addictive Behavior A-31

Chapter 12 Drinking Responsibly A-34

Chapter 13 Tobacco and Caffeine A-37

Chapter 14 Illicit Drugs A-40

Chapter 15 Cardiovascular Disease A-43

Chapter 16 Cancer A-46

Chapter 17 Infectious Diseases and Sexually Transmitted Infections A-49

Chapter 18 Noninfectious Conditions A-52

Chapter 19 Healthy Aging A-55

Chapter 20 Dying and Death A-58

Chapter 21 Environmental Health A-61

Chapter 22 Consumerism A-64

Chapter 23 Complementary and Alternative Medicine A-67

Appendix A: Injury Prevention and Emergency Care A-70

ANSWERS A-73

Preface

On the surface, the concept of taking charge of your health probably seems easy. But when put into practical terms, developing a personal and relevant plan of action can be difficult. It requires general health knowledge, the ability to critically assess yourself, and the discipline to set and follow through on personal goals. That's where this book can be of help to you. *Take Charge of Your Health* contains two distinct sections: a self-assessment workbook and a set of review and practice tests.

- The self-assessment guide, pages 1 to 191, can help you identify behavior patterns that affect your health status - both positively and negatively. Upon completion of each assessment, review the results and consider whether you need to make any adjustments in your health practices.
- The practice and review tests follow the self-assessment guide and are located on pages A-1 to A-83. This section includes two tests for each chapter that will assist you in the development of health knowledge. As you proceed through *Access to Health,* use the tests to check your retention of information.

Materials within the self-assessment and test sections correspond directly with the chapters in *Access to Health.* Use these materials in whichever way is most appropriate for your purposes, such as in preparation for upcoming exams. For greatest effectiveness, the following three-step model is recommended.

Step 1: Prior to beginning a chapter, complete the self-assessment exercises that apply to the chapter information and review the results to identify where attention may need to be placed. This will also help you identify content areas that need to be focused on during the course of study or areas that you may wish to explore further.

Step 2: After completing the reading and study of a chapter, take the corresponding practice and review tests and score your results.

Step 3: Once you have finished the chapter, review your completed self-assessment exercises and identify your strengths and weaknesses. Set goals for making improvements where necessary and consider strategies for attaining these goals. Your *Access to Health* text, including the Health Resource Guide in the book, can serve as a helpful resource for goal setting.

The exercises in *Take Charge of Your Health* can be used throughout your course of study and beyond. By using the self-assessments and practice and review tests provided in this workbook, you will be better equipped to truly "Take Charge" of your health.

Health Improvement Project

Name: Jennifer Lawrence Date: 9/13/10

Purpose: This health improvement project provides you with the opportunity to apply concepts covered in class toward improving any aspect of health. The project includes four steps:

Step 1 Assess your own health behaviors by completing Martin's Index of Health Behavior (1-2) and decide on a particular health behavior to be changed during the academic term.

Step 2 Complete the Health Improvement Contract (1-1a) to plan, guide, and evaluate your progress toward changing a specific habit that is detrimental to your health.

Step 3 Write an abstract of three separate journal articles that are pertinent to the behavior change. Your instructor can provide examples of current scholarly health journals that you might use for researching your area of interest. Each written abstract should include the following information:

1. Author, date published, title of article, name of journal, volume numbers, and pages.

2. Several paragraphs stating the main points of the article and conclusions reached if the article was a research report.

3. An evaluation of how this material will be helpful in validating or following through with the proposed behavior change. You should ask the question "Of what value is this information to me now or later in life?"

Step 4 Keep a journal and write two journal entries per week describing your progress and pitfalls as you work toward your personal goal. Include barriers encountered, successes, emotional and physical reactions to the changes, reactions of others to the changes, and your comments and feelings about the project. For some changes, a daily entry would be appropriate. The more seriously you treat your journal writing, the more you will benefit from this project.

Step 5 Write an evaluation of your health improvement project by answering the questions on form 1-1b.

HEALTH IMPROVEMENT CONTRACT

Name: Jennifer Lawrence Date: 9/14/10

Health habit or behavior I intend to change: eating habits (sugar intake); exercise habits

Goal to be reached (in specific terms): less sugar - more whole foods low in fat; exercise atleast 4-5 times or more per week

Current self-assessed status (refer to self-assessment scale from 1-2 Martin's Index of Health Behavior):
average but needing change

Benefits I anticipate as a result of the change:

(1) more energy
(2) more focus
(3) happier in general ♥

Any benefits of **not** changing?

(1) None!
(2)
(3)

What will happen if I don't change? become lethargic, lose sight of goals, become more negative in general

Specific activities, behaviors, attitudes, or thoughts I will monitor and chart during the 9-week period: indulgence, lack of drive, frustration levels, negative outlook, being down on myself, eating habits, activity level!

Target date to reach goal: 1 month (approx. 30 days) 10/14/10

Indicators of successful achievement of my health behavior change will be: reaching my goals, feeling better about myself and my situation, more energetic

How I will reward myself (daily, weekly, overall) for this change: Self praise, doing what it is I want in that moment

Names and phone numbers of HIP partners and times to meet to discuss progress: this is a journey of self realization therefor I will be my own judge!

Name: Jennifer Lawrence Date: 9/14/10

Signature

Instructor's signature

HEALTH IMPROVEMENT EVALUATION

Name: ______________________________ Date: ____________

1. Did you follow your plan? If so, did your timeline work? Were journal entries helpful? Were your support people valuable? If not, where did your plan break down? Was your goal unreasonable? What barriers hindered your progress?

Health Habit or Behavior: ______________________________

2. How do you feel about your efforts and any changes made?

3. How will you maintain your changed behavior?

MARTIN'S INDEX OF HEALTH BEHAVIOR

Name: Jennifer Lawrence Date: 9/14/10

Directions: For the following questions put a check in the blank by the choice that best describes your health behavior. There are no right or wrong answers. The best answer is the one that honestly describes you.

(1) 1. How many days per week do you eat breakfast?

___ a. 6-7 X c. 2-3

___ b. 4-5 ___ d. 0-1

(1) 2. Which choice most closely describes your daily eating pattern?

___ a. eating snack foods (potato chips, soda pop, etc.) whenever I am hungry

X b. eating one balanced meal per day and eating snack foods at other times during the day

___ c. eating two balanced meals a day and eating snack foods at other times of the day

___ d. eating three balanced meals a day and eating snack foods at other times of the day

___ e. eating three balanced meals per day and not snacking

(1) 3. How many days per week do you eat a balanced diet that includes the minimum number of servings from the four food groups as listed below?

2 servings of meat or protein substitutes
2 servings of dairy products
4 servings of breads and cereals
4 servings of fruits and vegetables

___ a. 6-7 X c. 2-3

___ b. 4-5 ___ d. 0-1

(2) 4. How many servings per day of concentrated sources of sugar (soda pop, candy, cookies, etc.) do you eat?

___ a. 0 or less than 1 ___ c. 3-4

X b. 1-2 ___ d. 5 or more

(2) 5. Considering your height and body build, how many pounds within your ideal weight do you fall?

___ a. within 10 pounds

X b. within 20 pounds

___ c. within 30 pounds

___ d. more than 30 pounds from ideal

(3) 6. Which choice most closely describes your dieting behavior?

___ a. never being overweight, so never dieting

___ b. being more than 10 pounds overweight, but not dieting

___ c. when overweight, going on a fad diet to lose weight quickly

___ d. when overweight, attempting to lose weight gradually (1-2 pounds per week) by increasing exercise *or* decreasing food intake

_X_ e. when overweight, attempting to lose weight gradually (1-2 pounds per week) by increasing exercise *and* decreasing food intake

(1) 7. What is the average number of hours per night that you sleep?

_X_ a. more than 10

___ b. 9-10

___ c. 7-8

___ d. 5-6

___ e. 0-4

(3) 8. How often do you use seatbelts while driving or riding in a car?

_X_ a. always

___ b. never in town and always on the highway

___ c. sometimes in town and sometimes on the highway

___ d. never

(2) 9. How often do you drive or ride with someone under the influence of alcohol or drugs?

___ a. more than once per week

___ b. once per week

_X_ c. a few times per year

___ d. never

(3) 10. Which choice best describes your consumption of alcoholic beverages?

_X_ a. not drinking

___ b. drinking one drink or less per day

___ c. drinking two drinks or less per day

___ d. drinking two drinks or less on weekdays, more than two drinks per day on weekends

___ e. drinking more than two drinks per day on most days

(1) 11. Which choice best describes your drug use patterns (over the counter, prescription, and recreational drugs)?

___ a. using the drugs I want whenever I want

_X_ b. using the drugs I feel I need while following common sense

___ c. using only medically required drugs exactly as directed

___ d. rarely using drugs of any kind

(2) 12. How many cups of caffeinated beverages (coffee, tea, cola, etc.) do you drink per day?

___ a. none or less than 1
X b. 1-3
___ c. 4-6
___ d. 7 or more

(3) 13. Which choice best describes your cigarette smoking behavior?

X a. not smoking
___ b. smoking less than one pack per day
___ c. smoking 1-2 packs per day
___ d. smoking more than 2 packs per day

(2) 14. How many times per week do you exercise aerobically (biking, jogging, swimming, aerobics, etc.)?

___ a. less than 1
___ b. 1
X c. 2
___ d. 3-4
___ e. 5 or more

(2) 15. How many times per week do you do other types of exercise (weight lifting, tennis, calisthenics, racquetball, basketball, etc.) besides aerobic activities?

___ a. less than 1
___ b. 1
X c. 2
___ d. 3-4
___ e. 5 or more

(1) 16. How often do you brush your teeth?

___ a. after every meal
___ b. twice per day
X c. once per day
___ d. less than once per day

(0) 17. How often do you have a dental check-up?

X a. never or only when something is wrong
___ b. every 2-3 years
___ c. every year
___ d. every six months

(1) 18. How often do you have a medical check-up?

___ a. never or only when something is wrong
X b. only for Pap tests or other checks
___ c. every 3-5 years
___ d. at least every 2 years

(1) 19. How often do you read the labels of foods and over-the-counter drugs before purchasing them?

___ a. always
___ b. usually
_X_ c. sometimes
___ d. rarely

(1) 20. How many times per week do you make a conscientious effort to manage your stress by utilizing progressive relaxation, exercise, religion, music, or other stress-reduction techniques?

___ a. 6-7
___ b. 4-5
_X_ c. 2-3
___ d. 0-1

(2) 21. Which choice most correctly describes your closest interpersonal relationship?

___ a. not having a friend
___ b. having a friend, but I am not able to share my real feelings with the person
_X_ c. having a friendship where I can sometimes share my real feelings, but sometimes can't
___ d. having a friendship where I can always share my real feelings

(2) 22. How many servings per day of foods high in saturated fats or cholesterol (whole milk, eggs, sausage, bacon, red meat, etc.) do you eat?

___ a. 0
_X_ b. 1-2
___ c. 3-4
___ d. 5 or more

(2) 23. How often do you limit your consumption of salt by doing things like not salting your foods at the table, using salt sparingly when preparing foods, and limiting your intake of salty foods?

___ a. always
_X_ b. usually
___ c. sometimes
___ d. rarely

(0) 24. How often do you practice breast self-examination (female) or testicular self-examination (male)?

___ a. every month
___ b. every 2-6 months
___ c. less frequently than every 6 months
_X_ d. never

25. Which choice best describes your contraceptive use?

___ a. not sexually active, so don't use contraceptives

___ b. attempting to get pregnant or am pregnant, so don't use contraceptives

___ c. sexually active and always use contraceptives

___ d. sexually active and usually use contraceptives

___ e. sexually active and sometimes use contraceptives

___ f. sexually active and rarely use contraceptives

Scoring:

For Items: 1, 3, 4, 5, 8, 12, 13, 16, 19, 20, 22, 23, 24
a=3, b=2, c=1, d=0

For Items: 2, 9, 11, 17, 18, 21
a=0, b=1, c=2, d=3

For Item: 6
a=3, b=1, c=0, d=2, e=3

For Item: 7
a=1, b=2, c=3, d=2, e=0

For Item: 10
a=3, b=3, c=2, 2=1, e=0

For Items: 14 and 15
a=0, b=1, c=2, d=3, e=3

For Item: 25
a=3, b=3, c=3, d=2, e=1, f=0

Total scores can range from 0-75. Health behavior is generally *poor* if the total score is below 25; *average but needing change* if between 25 and 50; and *good* if over 50.

Source: Joan Peterson Martin, The Relationship of Self Concept to Health Behavior in Community College Students (unpublished thesis). University of Chicago, December 1985.

Life Orientation Test

Name: ______________________________ Date: __________

Purpose: Do you see the cup as half full or half empty? Are you generally optimistic or pessimistic? Do you expect good things to happen or do you find the cloud around the silver lining? Optimism and pessimism are general expectations about what will happen to us--and how well we can influence what will happen to us--in the future. The Life Orientation Test may provide you with insight into whether you are basically optimistic or pessimistic in your outlook on life.

Directions: Indicate whether or not each of the items represents your feelings by writing a number in the blank space according to the following code. Then use the scoring key at the end of the test.

4 = strongly agree
3 = agree
2 = neutral
1 = disagree
0 = strongly disagree

___ 1. In uncertain times, I usually expect the best.

___ 2. It's easy for me to relax.

___ 3. If something can go wrong for me, it will.

___ 4. I always look on the bright side of things.

___ 5. I'm always optimistic about my future.

___ 6. I enjoy my friends a lot.

___ 7. It's important for me to keep busy.

___ 8. I hardly ever expect things to go my way.

___ 9. Things never work out the way I want them to.

___ 10. I don't get upset too easily.

___ 11. I'm a believer in the idea that "every cloud has a silver lining."

___ 12. I rarely count on good things happening to me.

Scoring: In order to arrive at your total score for the test, first reverse your score on items 3, 8, 9, and 12. That is, on those four items, 4 is changed to 0, 3 is changed to 1, 2 remains a 2, 1 is changed to 3, and 0 is changed to 4. Now add the numbers of items 1, 3, 4, 5, 8, 9, 11, and 12 (items 2, 6, 7, and 10 are "fillers" only, and your responses on them are not scored as part of the test. Your total score can vary from 0 to 32. Write your **total score here** ____.

Interpretation: Scheier and Carver (1985) provide the following norms for the test, based on administration to 357 undergraduate men and 267 undergraduate women. The average score for men was 21.03 (standard deviation = 4.56), and the average score for women was 21.41 (standard deviation = 5.22). The majority of undergraduates score between 16 and 26. Scores below 16 are quite pessimistic. Scores above 26 are quite optimistic.

Source: Michael F. Scheier and Charles S. Carver, 1985. Optimism, coping and health: Assessment and implications of generalized outcome expectancies. Health Psychology, 4, 219-247.

Multidimensional Health Locus of Control

Name: ____ Date: ____________

Directions: Indicate your degree of agreement with each statement by placing a number in the blank before it. Use the following scale:

5 = strongly agree
4 = agree
3 = neither agree nor disagree
2 = disagree
1 = strongly disagree

Subscale A: **Internal**

___ 1. If I get sick, it is my own behavior that determines how soon I get well.

___ 2. I am in control of my health.

___ 3. When I get sick, I am to blame.

___ 4. The main thing that affects my health is what I myself do.

___ 5. If I take care of myself, I can avoid illness.

___ 6. If I take the right actions, I can stay healthy.

Subscale B: **Powerful Others**

___ 1. Having regular contact with my physician is the best way for me to avoid illness.

___ 2. Whenever I don't feel well, I should consult a medically trained professional.

___ 3. My family has a lot to do with my becoming sick or staying healthy.

___ 4. Health professionals control my health.

___ 5. When I recover from an illness, it's usually because other people (e.g., doctors, nurses, family, and friends) have been taking good care of me.

___ 6. Regarding my health, I can only do what my doctor tells me to do.

Subscale C: **Chance**

___ 1. No matter what I do, if I am going to get sick, I will get sick.

___ 2. Most things that affect my health happen to me by accident.

___ 3. Luck plays a big part in determining how soon I will recover from an illness.

___ 4. My good health is largely a matter of good fortune.

___ 5. No matter what I do, I'm likely to get sick.

___ 6. If it's meant to be, I will stay healthy.

Scoring: To obtain your score for a subscale, add the numbers you chose in that subscale.

1. A score of 23-30 on any subscale means you have a strong inclination to that particular dimension. For example, a high C score would indicate you hold strong beliefs that your health is a matter of chance.

2. A score of 15-22 means you are moderate on that particular dimension. For example, a moderate B score would indicate you have moderate belief that your health is due to powerful others.

3. A score of 6-14 means you are low on that particular dimension. For example, a low A score means that you generally do not believe that you personally control your health

Interpretation: If you scored *high* on the internal health locus-of-control scale and low or moderate on the powerful others and chance scales, you are a person who feels that your health is basically under your control. If you scored *moderately* on the internal health locus-of-control, you are a person who feels that sometimes your health is under your control and sometimes it is not. For the moderately internal individual, the scores on the powerful others and chance scales would determine the relative weight on these other two dimensions.

If you scored *low* on the internal health locus-of-control scale, you are a person who feels that you do not have control over your own health. Your scores on the powerful others and chance scales would determine the relative influence of these other two dimensions. If you scored relatively high on the powerful others scale and moderate to low on the other two scales, you are a person who feels that powerful others (e.g., physicians) control your health. If you scored relatively high on the chance scale and moderate to low on the other two scales, you are a person who feels that chance, fate, or luck determines your health status.

Based on the Multidimensional Health Locus-of-Control Scales, you should have gained some insight into your perceptions of control over your health.

We neither have complete control nor lack of complete control over life outcomes. As we learn how to gain greater control over aspects of our environment, we will be able to make changes in stressful behaviors.

Getting Started: Self-Assessment

Name: ______________________________ Date: __________

Directions: Before you can begin to change negative patterns of behavior, you must determine where you are right now. Asking yourself the following questions should help you realistically take stock of your situation and start the process toward change.

1. *What would I* most like to change about myself right now?

2. *What do I* believe about the impact of this behavior on my health right now?

Severity:

Susceptibility:

Benefit to be derived vs. cost to me:

Likelihood of success:

3. *Who am I trying to please* by changing this behavior? Who is influencing me to do it? Why?

4. *What* positive reinforcing, predisposing, and enabling factors will help me achieve my goals?

Reinforcing:

Predisposing:

Enabling:

5. *What* negative reinforcing, predisposing, and enabling factors will stand in the way of my achieving my goals?

Reinforcing:

Predisposing:

Enabling:

6. *Can I do anything* to reduce the impact or alter the negative factors?

7. *What actions will I take to get started?*

What Health Screening Examinations Do You Need?

Directions: Circle the appropriate response.

Yes	No	1.	Do you have diabetes?
Yes	No	2.	Are you over age 40 and African American?
Yes	No	3.	Are you over are over age 60?
Yes	No	4.	Have you had sexual intercourse without condoms?
Yes	No	5.	Have you had multiple sexual partners?
Yes	No	6.	Have you had a sexually transmitted disease?
Yes	No	7.	Have you injected illegal drugs or had a blood transfusion between 1978 and 1985?
Yes	No	8.	Have you had a family member with diabetes?
Yes	No	9.	Are you overweight?
Yes	No	10.	Have you had diabetes during pregnancy:
Yes	No	11.	Are over age 65?
Yes	No	12.	Now or in the past, have you ever consumed a lot of alcohol or
Yes	No	13.	Now or in the past, have you smoked or chewed tobacco:
Yes	No	14.	Are you a man 50 years of age or older?
Yes	No	15.	Are you a man aged 18-35 years (particularly if you have a testicle that is abnormally small or not in the normal position)?
Yes	No	16.	Have you had skin cancer in your family?
Yes	No	17.	Have you had a lot of sun exposure?
Yes	No	18.	Have you had radiation treatments of your upper body?
Yes	No	19.	Have you been exposed to tuberculosis (TB)?
Yes	No	20.	Have you recently moved from Asia, Africa, Central or South America, or the Pacific Islands?
Yes	No	21.	Have you had kidney failure, diabetes, HIV, or alcoholism?
Yes	No	22.	Do you use illegal drugs?
Yes	No	23.	Are you a woman 50 years of age or older?
Yes	No	24.	Are you a woman 18 years of age older?

Scoring

If you answer "Yes" to any of the statements, discuss whether you need a health or medical screening with your health-care provider. Use the Personal Information Form and Personal Preventive Record on the following pages to track your preventive care.

If you answered "Yes" to questions:	Type of exam you may need
1 – 3	routine eye examinations.
4 – 7	AIDS (HIV), syphilis, gonorrhea, chlamydia, or hepatitis
8 – 10	diabetes (glucose) test.
11	hearing test.
12 – 13	mouth examination.
14	prostate examination.
15	testicular examination.
16 – 17	skin examination.
18	thyroid examination.
19 –22	tuberculosis test.
23	mammogram.
24	Pap smear and gynecological examination.

Source: Adapted from the April 1998, Publication *Personal Health Guide: Put Prevention into Practice.* Consumer Information. Agency for Health Care Policy and Research, Rockville, MD.

Personal Information Form

Staying on top of your health history can be challenging. The records in this Guide can help you keep track of information. These records will be especially useful to you whenever you visit your health care provider or should you become incapacitation. First, record your background information here. You can access other records for preventive tests, vaccinations, exams, additional preventive care measures, and medications.

Name:____

Address: ____

Telephone: ____

In an emergency, contact:

____

Allergies: ____

____

Health care provider name(s) and phone number(s):

____

____

Medical insurance name(s) and number(s): ____________________________

____

Personal Prevention Record

Use this Personal Prevention Record to keep track of the preventive care that you have received and/or will need in the future. With the help of your health care provider, fill in how often you need each type of preventive care. Write in the date each time you receive preventive care. Use the remaining space to record other information (such as results of tests and the health care provider's or clinic's name). Use the records for Additional Preventive Care, and Medication to keep track of other important medical information.

Type of Preventive Care	Dates	Information	Results	Goal	Routine Schedule
Blood pressure					
Cholesterol					
Weight					
Fecal occult blood test					
Sigmoidoscopy					
Tetanus (Td) shot					Every 10 years
Pneumococcal shot					Once at age 65
Influenza shot					Every year starting at age 65
Dental visits					At least yearly

Medication Record

Write down each medicine you take, the reason you take it, and how you take it.
Also include any over-the-counter medicines, such as:

Laxatives
Diet pills
Vitamins
Cold medicine
Aspirin or other pain, headache, or fever medicine
Cough medicine
Allergy relief medicine
Antacids
Sleeping pills
Others (include names)

Medication Name	Dose	How Often	Time of Day	Reason Taken	How Taken (e.g., before meals)

Develop Your Own Support System

Name: ______________________________ Date: __________

We all need different kinds of friends. Different friends are able to complement the different aspects of our personalities. For instance, we may have some friends with whom we are silly and other friends with whom we are more serious. One person cannot possibly fill all the needs we have in friends, so we must look for more.

The following suggestions are designed to help you build or improve your social support system.

1. Look for different qualities in different people.
2. Accept and enjoy what others have to offer.
3. Accept that others have limitations.
4. Offer only what you are willing to give.
5. Realize that your time and your friendship are precious.

Keep a written record of the names and roles of your social support system below.

Person:	How this person might help:
________________________	________________________
________________________	________________________
________________________	________________________
________________________	________________________
________________________	________________________
________________________	________________________
________________________	________________________
________________________	________________________

Health center phone number: ____________________

Self-Esteem Inventory - Part I

Name: ______________________ Date: ____________

Purpose: The Self-Esteem Inventory will help you determine attitudes you have toward yourself. Such attitudes are an important part of emotional well-being.

Directions: Read each statement. Then decide if you strongly agree, agree disagree, or strongly disagree with the statement. Circle the number in the column that corresponds to your response.

	Strongly Agree	Agree	Disagree	Strongly Disagree
1. I feel that I'm a person of worth, at least on an equal plane with others.	4	3	2	1
2. I feel that I have a number of good qualities.	4	3	2	1
3. All in all, I am inclined to feel that I am a failure.	1	2	3	4
4. I am able to do things as well as most other people.	4	3	2	1
5. I feel I do not have as much to be proud of as others.	1	2	3	4
6. I take a positive attitude toward myself.	4	3	2	1
7. On the whole, I am satisfied with myself.	4	3	2	1
8. I wish I could have more respect for myself.	1	2	3	4
9. I certainly feel useless at times.	1	2	3	4
10. At times I think I am no good at all.	1	2	3	4

Scoring: Add *all* the numbers you circled. Then divide the total by 10.

Total ________ divided by 10 = __________

Interpretation:

4.0 = Highest self-esteem level
3.5-3.9 = High self-esteem
3.0-3.4 = Above-average self-esteem
2.0-2.9 = Below-average self-esteem
< 2.0 = Low self-esteem

Source: Peggy Blake, Robert Frye, and Michael Pejsach, Discover Your Health Behaviors. New York: Random House, 1987.

Self-Esteem Inventory - Part II Personal Application

Name: ______________________________ Date: __________

Purpose: Becoming aware of positive qualities and attributes increases self- esteem.

List 10 of your positive qualities.

1. ______________________________
2. ______________________________
3. ______________________________
4. ______________________________
5. ______________________________
6. ______________________________
7. ______________________________
8. ______________________________
9. ______________________________
10. ______________________________

o If you were to die in the next hour, what good characteristics would people remember about you? Write a eulogy for yourself.

- o Think about a person in your life whom you greatly respect. What causes you to respect that person? How are *you* similar or different? How could you emphasize qualities about yourself that are similar to those of the respected person? How could you change those aspects of you that are dissimilar?

- o You affect other people's self-esteem. Think of someone with whom you regularly spend time. What do you do to improve his or her self-esteem?

Source: Peggy Blake, Robert Frye, and Michael Pejsach, Discover Your Health Behaviors. New York: Random House, 1987.

Need for Uniqueness Scale

Name: ______________________________________ Date: ____________

Directions: The following statements concern your perceptions about yourself in a variety of situations. Your task is to indicate the strength of your agreement with each statement utilizing a scale in which 1 denotes strong disagreement, 5 denotes strong agreement, and 2, 3, and 4 represent intermediate judgments. In the blank preceding each statement, place your number from *1 to 5. There are no "right" or "wrong" answers, so select the number that most clearly reflects you on each statement.*

__ 1. When I am in a group of strangers, I am not reluctant to express my opinion openly.

__ 2. I find that criticism affects my self-esteem.

__ 3. I sometimes hesitate to use my own ideas for fear they might be impractical.

__ 4. I think society should let reason lead it to new customs and throw aside old habits or mere traditions.

__ 5. People frequently succeed in changing my mind.

__ 6. I find it sometimes amusing to upset the dignity of teachers, judges, and "cultured" people.

__ 7. I like wearing a uniform because it makes me proud to be a member of the organization it represents.

__ 8. People have sometimes called me "stuck-up."

__ 9. Others' disagreements make me uncomfortable.

__ 10. I do not always need to live by the rules and standards of society.

__ 11. I am unable to express my feelings if they result in undesirable consequences.

__ 12. Being a success in one's career means making a contribution that no one else has made.

__ 13. It bothers me if people think I am being too unconventional.

__ 14. I always try to follow rules.

__ 15. If I disagree with a superior on his or her views, I usually do not keep it to myself.

__ 16. I speak up in meetings in order to oppose those whom I feel are wrong.

__ 17. Feeling "different" in a crowd of people makes me feel uncomfortable.

__ 18. If I must die, let it be an unusual death rather than an ordinary death in bed.

__ 19. I would rather be just like everyone else than be called a "freak."

__ 20. I must admit I find it hard to work under strict rules and regulations.

__ 21. I would rather be known for always trying new ideas than for employing well-trusted methods.

__ 22. It is better always to agree with the opinions of others than to be considered a disagreeable person.

__ 23. I do not like to say unusual things to people.

__ 24. I tend to express my opinions publicly, regardless of what others say.

__ 25. As a rule, I strongly defend my own opinions.

__ 26. I do not like to go my own way.

__ 27. When I am with a group of people, I agree with their ideas so that no arguments will arise.

__ 28. I tend to keep quiet in the presence of persons of higher rank, experience, etc.

__ 29. I have been quite independent and free from family rule.

__ 30. Whenever I take part in group activities, I am somewhat of a non-conformist.

__ 31. In most things in life, I believe in playing it safe rather than taking a gamble.

__ 32. It is better to break rules than always to conform with an impersonal society.

Scoring: Reverse score on items 2, 3, 5, 7, 9, 11, 13, 14, 17, 19, 22, 23, 26, 27, 28, and 31. On these items, a 5=1, 4=2, 3=3, 2=4, and 1=5. Then add the score for all 32 items. The *higher* the score, the greater the *need for uniqueness*. The scale does not necessarily tell how different one actually is. Of 1400 students at the University of Kansas and Purdue University, a score of 100 was the 50th percentile.

Source: C.R. Snyder and H.L. Fromkin. 1980 Uniqueness: The human pursuit of difference. New York: Plenum Press, pp. 79-80.

Self-Actualization Inventory

Name: ______________________________ Date: __________

Purpose: To make you aware of the characteristics of self-actualization. Also, to help you find out whether you are a self-actualizing person; that is, a person who is fulfilling his or her potentials, including esthetic, creative, and spiritual capacities.

Directions: Circle the number in the column on the right side that you feel honestly describes how you feel or behave.

Characteristics	Frequency: Very Often	Often	Sometimes	Never
1. Judge others accurately	5	3	1	0
2. Detect falseness in others	5	3	1	0
3. Tolerate uncertainty	5	3	1	0
4. Accept your good and bad aspects	5	3	1	0
5. Accept others even though you disagree with them	5	3	1	0
6. Get creative ideas	5	3	1	0
7. Enjoy doing unplanned and unrehearsed things	15	10	4	0
8. Involved with problems of others	10	7	3	0
9. Able to be alone (by yourself)	10	7	3	0
10. Able to be honest self when with strangers	5	3	1	0
11. Resist local customs and traditions	5	3	1	0
12. Have your friends support you before making decisions	5	3	1	0
13. Able to make decisions	5	3	1	0
14. Get a lot of enjoyment from playing or socializing with others	5	3	1	0
15. Appreciate seeing a play or concert	5	3	1	0
16. Feel inspired after hearing or seeing outstanding artists/persons perform	5	3	1	0
17. Have empathy for how another person feels	5	3	1	0
18. Help others to grow and become better persons	5	3	1	0
19. Have deep and meaningful relationships with a few friends	5	3	1	0
20. Feel that a person should be hired on ability and competency	5	3	1	0
21. Do work that you enjoy	10	7	3	0
22. Feel that your work is important	5	3	1	0
23. Laugh at yourself	10	7	3	0
24. Look forward to new experiences	10	7	3	0
25. Enjoy peak and unusual experiences	15	12	4	0
26. Believe that honesty is the best policy	5	3	1	0
27. Believe that one should always tell the truth	5	3	1	0
28. Have dedication to life or social purpose	10	7	3	0

Total ______________

Scoring: Add the numbers you circled. This is your self-actualization score. Classify your score in the appropriate score range.

Score Range	Current potential for self-actualization
150-200	High self-actualization
112-149	Moderate self-actualization
80-111	Approaching self-actualization
0-79	Below average self-actualization

Source: Walter D. Sorochan. Personal Health Appraisal. New York: Wiley & Sons, Publishers, 1976, 37-40.

How Hardy Are You?

Name: ____________________________________ Date: ____________

Purpose: Below are 12 items similar to those that appear in the hardiness questionnaire. Evaluating someone's hardiness requires more than this quick test. But this simple exercise should give you some idea of how hardy you are.

Directions: Write down how much you agree or disagree with the following statements, using this scale:

0 = strongly disagree
1 = mildly disagree
2 = mildly agree
3 = strongly agree

___ A. Trying my best at work makes a difference.

___ B. Trusting to fate is sometimes all I can do in a relationship.

___ C. I often wake up eager to start on the day's projects.

___ D. Thinking of myself as a free person leads to great frustration and difficulty.

___ E. I would be willing to sacrifice financial security in my work if something really challenging came along.

___ F. It bothers me when I have to deviate from the routine or schedule I've set for myself.

___ G. An average citizen can have an impact on politics.

___ H. Without the right breaks, it is hard to be successful in my field.

___ I. I know why I am doing what I'm doing at work.

___ J. Getting close to people puts me at risk of being obligated to them.

___ K. Encountering new situations is an important priority in my life.

___ L. I really don't mind when I have nothing to do.

Scoring: These questions measure control, commitment and challenge. For half the questions, a high score (like 3,"strongly agree") indicates hardiness; for the other half, a low score (disagreement) does.

To get your scores on control, commitment and challenge, first write in the number of your answer-0,1,2 to 3-above the letter of each question on the score sheet. Then add and subtract as shown. (To get your score on "control", for example, add your answers to question A and G; add your answers to B and H; and then subtract the second number from the first.)

Add your scores on commitment, control and challenge together to get a score for total hardiness.

A total score of **10-18** shows a hardy personality, **0-9** moderate hardiness. Below **0** low hardiness.

___ + ___ = ___	___ + ___ = ___	___ + ___ = ___
A G	C I	E K
___ + ___ = ___	___ + ___ = ___	___ + ___ = ___
B H Control Score	D J Commitment Score	F L Challenge Score

________ + ________ + ________ = ________

Control + Commitment + Challenge = Total Hardiness Score

Source: Joan Luckman, Your Health. Englewood Cliffs, NJ: Prentice Hall, 1991.

Inventory of Negative Thoughts

Name: ______________________________ Date: __________

Purpose: Cognitive theorists believe that people can make themselves depressed by thinking negative thoughts. The following inventory includes many negative thoughts that are commonly linked to depression. How many of them have you experienced in recent months? Do they strike you as accurate and appropriate to your situation? Or are you giving in to cognitive distortions that can lead to feelings of depression?

Directions: Using the code below, write in a number from 1 to 4 to indicate how frequently you have the thoughts contained in the list that follows. Pay particular attention to the content of the thought rather than the specific wording.

1. Never 2. Seldom 3. Often 4. Very Often

___ 1. It seems such an effort to do anything.
___ 2. I feel pessimistic about the future.
___ 3. I have too many bad things in my life.
___ 4. I have very little to look forward to.
___ 5. I'm drained of energy, worn out.
___ 6. I'm not as successful as other people.
___ 7. Everything seems futile and pointless.
___ 8. I just want to curl up and go to sleep.
___ 9. There are things about me that I don't like.
___ 10. It's too much effort even to move.
___ 11. I'm absolutely exhausted.
___ 12. The future seems just one string of problems.
___ 13. My thoughts keep drifting away.
___ 14. I get no satisfaction from the things I do.
___ 15. I've made so many mistakes in the past.
___ 16. I've got to really concentrate just to keep my eyes open.
___ 17. Everything I do turns out badly.
___ 18. My whole body has slowed down.
___ 19. I regret some of the things I've done.
___ 20. I can't make the effort to liven up myself.
___ 21. I feel depressed with the way things are going.
___ 22. I haven't any real friends anymore.
___ 23. I do have a number of problems.
___ 24. There's no one I can feel really close to.

___ 25. I wish I were someone else.

___ 26. I'm annoyed at myself for being bad at making decisions.

___ 27. I don't make a good impression on other people.

___ 28. The future look hopeless.

___ 29. I don't get the same satisfaction out of things these days.

___ 30. I wish something would happen to make me feel better.

Assertiveness Scale

Name: ______________________________________ Date: ____________

Purpose: This inventory is designed to give you an indication of your own degree of assertiveness.

Directions: Respond to each statement by circling the letter that best represents how you would generally respond in the given situation. If the situation does not apply to you, respond according to what you think would best characterize your behavior. Keep in mind that your responses should be your honest opinion of what you actually do or would do in these situations, not what you wish you could do.

Response Scale:	A	B	C	D	E
	Never	Rarely	Sometimes	Often	Always

1. In conversation I find it difficult to maintain eye contact.
   Never A B C D E Always
2. When I meet new people in situations, I initiate introductions and start conversations.
   Never A B C D E Always
3. My close friends dominate decisions about how we spend our leisure time together.
   Never A B C D E Always
4. If I am angry with friends/parents/roommates, I find it difficult to directly communicate my feelings to them.
   Never A B C D E Always
5. I ignore it when someone cuts in line in front of me.
   Never A B C D E Always
6. When a friend or roommate is overdue in returning something valuable, I mention it.
   Never A B C D E Always
7. If someone were tapping my chair in class or constantly talking during a movie, I would ask them to stop.
   Never A B C D E Always
8. I feel comfortable asking reasonable favors of other people.
   Never A B C D E Always
9. When family or friends, I find it difficult to break into or even initiate a conversation.
   Never A B C D E Always
10. If someone's cigarette smoke were bothering me in a public building I would politely ask them to stop.
    Never A B C D E Always
11. In regard to necessary chores, I insist that a roommate or partner take on a fair share.
    Never A B C D E Always

Response Scale:	A	B	C	D	E
	Never	Rarely	Sometimes	Often	Always

12. I avoid asking questions in class fearing that they just won't sound right.
Never A B C D E Always

13. If my instructor made, in my opinion, an unfair request, I would express my feelings to him or her.

14. I will buy things I really don't need if a salesman applies pressure.
Never A B C D E Always

15. If my dinner in a restaurant were not to my liking, I would demand that it be corrected.
Never A B C D E Always

16. I feel uncomfortable when someone give me a compliment.
Never A B C D E Always

17. I would freely offer information or my opinion in group discussions, even if I didn't know the other people very well.
Never A B C D E Always

18. I have difficulty communicating with an attractive person of the opposite sex.
Never A B C D E Always

19. I feel uncomfortable about returning a defective piece of merchandise.
Never A B C D E Always

20. I would be reluctant to invite someone of the opposite sex out on a date.
Never A B C D E Always

21. I would feel uncomfortable explaining to a friend/boss/instructor a better way, in my opinion, of completing a specific task.
Never A B C D E Always

Scoring: Use the following table to determine the number of points to assign to each of your responses. To determine your total score, add all the numbers that match the letter (A,B,C,D, or E) you circled for each statement.

Statement	A	B	C	D	E
1.	4	3	2	1	0
2.	0	1	2	3	4
3.	4	3	2	1	0
4.	4	3	2	1	0
5.	4	3	2	1	0
6.	0	1	2	3	4
7.	0	1	2	3	4
8.	0	1	2	3	4

Statement	A	B	C	D	E
9.	4	3	2	1	0
10.	0	1	2	3	4
11.	0	1	2	3	4
12.	4	3	2	1	0
13.	0	1	2	3	4
14.	4	3	2	1	0
15.	0	1	2	3	4
16.	0	1	2	3	4
17.	0	1	2	3	4
18.	4	3	2	1	0
19.	4	3	2	1	0
20.	4	3	2	1	0
21.	4	3	2	1	0

Total Score ______ This is your assertiveness score. Classify your score in the appropriate level.

66-84	Very Assertive
44-65	Somewhat Assertive
22-43	Somewhat Unassertive
0-21	Very Unassertive

Interpretation: Assertiveness is different from both passiveness and aggressiveness. It is not, as some people might think, halfway between these; it is quite different. Passiveness refers to acquiescing to another person's demands regardless of the consequences to yourself. Aggressiveness means attempting to force your desires on another person in order to satisfy your own needs, regardless of the other person's rights. Assertiveness is characterized by a degree of confidence in your pursuits combined with respect for your fellow human beings-respect that you would expect in a reciprocating manner. With each of the situations listed, an aggressive statement or assertive statement could be made. Keep in mind that assertiveness is determined not only be the words stated, but also in the tone of voice and body language. In addition, the individual on the receiving end of a statement may perceive the circumstances of statement differently and therefore view what was intended to be assertive as an aggressive act.

Source: Sandra Kammerman et al, Wellness RSVP. Menlo Park, CA: Benjamin Cummings, 1993. 47-49.

Could You Have Panic Disorder?

Answer the following questions to find out whether or not you may have panic disorder.

Yes No Do you experience sudden episodes of intense and overwhelming fear that seem to come on for no apparent reason?

Yes No During these episodes, do you also experience several of the following symptoms?

- Racing, pounding, or skipping heartbeat
- Chest pain, pressure, or discomfort
- Difficulty catching your breath
- Choking sensation or lump in your throat
- Excessive sweating
- Lightheadedness or dizziness
- Nausea or stomach problems
- Tingling or numbness in parts of your body
- Chills or hot flashes
- Shaking or trembling
- Feelings of unreality, or being detached from your body

Yes No During these episodes, do you have the urge to flee, or the feeling that you need to escape?

Yes No During these episodes, do you think something terrible might happen--that you might die, have a heart attack, suffocate, lose control, or embarrass yourself?

Yes No Do you worry a lot about these episodes or fear that they will happen again?

Yes No Does this fear cause you to avoid places or situations that you think might have triggered the attack?

Scoring
If you answered "Yes" to most of these questions, you may be suffering from panic disorder. This checklist is designed for educational purposes only. The information contained herein is not intended to substitute for informed medical advice or training. You should not use this information to diagnose or treat a mental health problem without consulting a qualified health or mental health care provider.

Source: July 1997 Healthwise Newsletter, National Institutes of Health

Anxiety Symptoms Checklist

Directions: Indicate whether or not you experience any of these symptoms.

Yes	No	Are you always worried about things even when there are no signs of trouble?
Yes	No	Do you seem unable to relax?
Yes	No	Do you often have trouble falling or staying asleep?
Yes	No	Are your worries accompanied by physical symptoms, especially trembling, twitching, muscle tension, headaches, irritability, sweating, or hot flashes?
Yes	No	Do you frequently feel lightheaded or out of breath?
Yes	No	Do you startle more easily than other people?
Yes	No	Do you tend to have trouble concentrating?
Yes	No	Is your body constantly tense?
Yes	No	Do you get tired easily, yet have trouble sleeping?
Yes	No	Do you have frequent aches and pains that cannot be traced to physical illness or injury?

Scoring

For every question you answered "Yes" you have indicated that you experience a symptom of Generalized Anxiety Disorder. If several of these symptoms seem to last for as long as 6 months, you may want to consult a mental health care provider about the possibility of having an anxiety disorder.

This checklist is designed for educational purposes only. The information contained herein is not intended to substitute for informed medical advice or training. You should not use this information to diagnose or treat a mental health problem without consulting a qualified health or mental health care provider.

Source: National Institutes of Mental Health, National Institutes of Health, Printed 1994, Reprinted 1995, 1997

Satisfaction with Life Scale

Directions

Below are five statements with which you may agree or disagree. Using the scale below indicate your level of agreement with each item by placing the appropriate number on the line preceding that item. Please be open and honest in your responses.

7 - Strongly agree
6 - Agree
5 - Slightly agree
4 - Neither agree or disagree
3 - Slightly disagree
2 - Disagree
1 - Strongly disagree

_____ In most ways my life is close to my ideal.

_____ The conditions of my life are excellent.

_____ I am satisfied with my life.

_____ So far I have gotten the important things I want in life.

_____ If I could live my life over, I would change almost nothing.

Scoring

The Satisfaction With Life Scale (SWLS) was developed to assess satisfaction with the respondent's life as a whole. The score is the combined total of the answers to the five statements.

35 - 31 Extremely satisfied
26 - 30 Satisfied
21 - 25 Slightly satisfied
20 Neutral
15 - 19 Slightly dissatisfied
10 - 14 Dissatisfied
5 - 9 Extremely dissatisfied

Source: The Satisfaction With Life Scale was developed by Ed Diener in 1984. *Journal of Personality Assessment* Vol.49 No.1 1985

People in Your Life

Directions: This survey is about the support and assistance people may receive from others. Using the following scale, for each item use a check (✓) to show how sure you are that you receive the kind of support described.

Definitely Yes = DY
Probably Yes = PY
Maybe = M
Probably No = PN
Definitely No = DN

DY	PY	M	PN	DN	
					1. Are there people you trust to give you advice?
					2. Are there people you feel comfortable contacting if you are lonely?
					3. Are there people who would go out of their way to give you a ride if you needed one?
					4. Are there people who would look after your home if you went away for awhile?
					5. Are there people who are willing to criticize you for your own good?
					6. Are there people who are proud of your accomplishments?
					7. Are there people who would help you move to a new home?
					8. Are there people who would lend you money if you needed it?
					9. Are there people with whom you share your deepest thoughts and feelings?
					10. Are there people who would help you if you had too much to do?
					11. Are there people you could stay with if you needed to get away for awhile?
					12. Are there people who help you feel good about yourself?
					13. Are there people who caredeeply about you?

DY	PY	M	PN	DN	
					14. Are there people you call if you want to go out on the spur of the moment?
					15. Are there people who would run errands for you if you were sick?
					16. Are there people who accept you just the way you are?
					17. Are there people who give you physical affection?
					18. Are there people who are willing to help you make important decisions?
					19. Are there people who help you feel better when you are upset?
					20. Are there people who help you work out personal problems?
					21. Are there people who are supportive of you no matter what?

Scoring

Point values are assigned to responses as follows:

Definitely Yes = 5
Probably Yes = 4
Maybe = 3
Probably No = 2
Definitely No = 1

Your Total Score: _______

This inventory can be scored by adding the point values of all responses and dividing this total by the number of responses (21). Blank items should not be counted in the number of responses. The maximum attainable score of 5 points indicates a high level of perceived social support. A minimum score of 1 suggests very weak perceived social support. This affective measure assesses your perceived support and assistance from people around you. Information about your perceived support from other people can be used to determine if you need assistance in strengthening your support network.

Source: Adapted from CDC, *Program Evaluation Handbook: Stress Management*, 1988, IOX Assessment Associates.

Assessing and Managing Stress
Part I: Stress Danger Signals

Name: ______________________________ Date: ____________

Purpose: The danger signals listed below focus on the medical and physical symptoms common to tension stress. Your physician can make the best determination of your medical condition, of course, but these guidelines can provide a rough measure of your stress level.

Directions: Check the signals you have.

___ 1. General irritability, hyperexcitation, or depression.

___ 2. Pounding of the heart.

___ 3. Dryness of mouth and throat.

___ 4. Impulsive behavior, emotional instability.

___ 5. Overpowering urge to cry or run or hide.

___ 6. Inability to concentrate, flight of thoughts, disorientation.

___ 7. Feelings of unreality, weakness, dizziness.

___ 8. Fatigue.

___ 9. Floating anxiety, being afraid and not knowing why.

___ 10. Emotional tension and alertness: "keyed up."

___ 11. Trembling, nervous.

___ 12. Tendency to be easily startled by small sounds.

___ 13. High pitched, nervous laughter.

___ 14. Stuttering, other speech difficulties.

___ 15. Bruxism, or grinding of teeth.

___ 16. Insomnia.

___ 17. Hypermotility, an increased tendency to move about without any reason.

___ 18. Sweating.

___ 19. Frequent need to urinate.

___ 20. Diarrhea, indigestion, queasiness in the stomach, and sometime vomiting.

___ 21. Migraine headaches.

___ 22. Pain in the neck and lower back.

___ 23. Loss of appetite or excessive appetite.

___ 24. Increased smoking.

___ 25. Increased use of prescribed drugs.

___ 26. Alcohol and drug abuse.

___ 27. Nightmares

___ 28. Accident proneness.

Interpretation: The more signs that are present, the stronger the likelihood that there is a serious problem.

Part II: Monitoring Events and Reactions

Directions: Monitor specific events that trigger stress by keeping a stress journal to record not only events but emotional, physical, and behavioral reactions. The following is just one format for recording this information:

	Time of day	Reactions (physical and emotional)	Stressor (situation, event)
Monday			
Tuesday			
Wednesday			
Thursday			
Friday			
Saturday			
Sunday			

Part III: Stress Management

After identifying stressful events, you may choose to attend a college or community-sponsored stress management workshop, or construct your own stress management plans. In developing a stress-management plan, consider the following:

- Time management/establishing priorities.
- Improvement in nutrition and eating habits.
- Aerobic exercise.
- Cognitive measure (for example, autogenics, visualization, and affirmations).
- Relaxation techniques--for example, progressive relaxation, massage and music. (See 5-3.)
- Pleasure.

A Time Management Questionnaire for College Students

Name: ______________________________ Date: ____________

Response Scale:	Never	Sometimes	Often	Almost Always
	0	+1	+2	+3

Planning

1. I keep in writing my short-term and long-term professional and personal goals.
   Never 0 +1 +2 +3 Almost always
2. I update in writing my professional and personal goals.
   Never 0 +1 +2 +3 Almost always
3. At the start of a semester I record all dates and due dates for exams, term papers, etc., in my planning calendar.
   Never 0 +1 +2 +3 Almost always
4. I write out my daily activities on a to-do list.
   Never 0 +1 +2 +3 Almost always
5. I prioritize the items on my to-do list and make sure that the priority items are done.
   Never 0 +1 +2 +3 Almost always
6. I schedule my most important work to occur during my "most alert" or "peak energy" hours.
   Never 0 +1 +2 +3 Almost always

My Desk and/or Study Area

7. My desk top is clean and contains only the project on which I'm currently working.
   Never 0 +1 +2 +3 Almost always
8. I get a positive feeling when I approach my desk.
   Never 0 +1 +2 +3 Almost always
9. I have a well-organized place for everything (books, notebooks, etc.).
   Never 0 +1 +2 +3 Almost always
10. I put everything in its place.
    Never 0 +1 +2 +3 Almost always
11. I can easily find items in my work area when I look for them.
    Never 0 +1 +2 +3 Almost always
12. My work space is well-lit, quiet, and conducive to good work.
    Never 0 +1 +2 +3 Almost always
13. I use a formal sign-out system for keeping track of books and other items that I lend to others.
    Never 0 +1 +2 +3 Almost always

Obtaining Results

14. I plan ahead and set reasonable deadlines for myself concerning studying, term projects, etc.
Never 0 +1 +2 +3 Almost always

15. I begin and finish projects on time and meet my deadlines.
Never 0 +1 +2 +3 Almost always

16. I concentrate on one task at a time.
Never 0 +1 +2 +3 Almost always

17. I perform time-consuming projects in short steps or stages.
Never 0 +1 +2 +3 Almost always

18. When going to meetings or appointments, I always have something with me to read to take advantage of "waiting" time.
Never 0 +1 +2 +3 Almost always

Time Savers Involving Myself and Others

19. I try to arrange nonacademic activities and meetings during my "least alert" times (For most students, these times are late in the afternoon and late in the evening.)
Never 0 +1 +2 +3 Almost always

20. I politely resist requests from my friends to socialize or have coffee during my scheduled study time and especially during my "most alert" time.
Never 0 +1 +2 +3 Almost always

21. When doing a project with another student, I set appointments so that we can review a number of items at one time.
Never 0 +1 +2 +3 Almost always

22. When having coffee or socializing with friends during a study break, I suggest *at the start* of the break that we agree on a time to get back to studying, and I stick to our agreement.
Never 0 +1 +2 +3 Almost always

23. I am politely assertive about cutting off long-winded telephone callers and/or other instances where people just want to "shoot the breeze."
Never 0 +1 +2 +3 Almost always

Scoring: To score the Time Management Questionnaire, add your points together and compare yourself with the scale below.

Interpretation:

50-69 You already manage your time very well.

35-49 You are on your way to being an effective time manager. However, you should increase the frequency with which you follow various time-saving strategies.

20-34 There is definite room for improvement in your time management skills. You need to take formal steps to implement some of the recommendations in this chapter in order to put more time into your life.

0-19 You're disorganized, overwhelmed, and spending far too much time on low-priority activities and time wasters. Take immediate steps to implement some of the recommendations in this chapter.

How Do You Handle Conflict?

Name: ______________________________________ Date: ____________

Purpose: It can be stated with confidence that people will face conflict throughout their lives. Dealing with conflict effectively is an important factor in human dynamics. There are different ways of dealing with conflict. This exercise will help you identify the methods you use.

Directions: The following statements describe possible responses to various conflict situations. Read each statement carefully, and circle the number on the scale below each statement that most closely describes your behavior.

Response Scale:	1	2	3	4	5
	Never	Rarely	Sometimes	Often	Always

1. When strong conflict occurs, I prefer to leave the situation.
   Never 1 2 3 4 5 Always
2. I feel very comfortable about taking a conflict between a friend and me to a third person.
   Never 1 2 3 4 5 Always
3. I try to find a compromise when a conflict occurs.
   Never 1 2 3 4 5 Always
4. I find conflict exciting and challenging.
   Never 1 2 3 4 5 Always
5. I tend to concentrate on the problem and the issues in a conflict rather than the other person.
   Never 1 2 3 4 5 Always
6. When conflict occurs, I act as though there is no real problem and try to "get along."
   Never 1 2 3 4 5 Always
7. I prefer to have a third person help solve a conflict between a friend and me.
   Never 1 2 3 4 5 Always
8. I'm willing to give a little if the other person in a dispute is also willing to give on some things.
   Never 1 2 3 4 5 Always
9. It's important that I win, even if the problem or issue in a disagreement is not really important to me.
   Never 1 2 3 4 5 Always
10. I search for a solution to a conflict that both the other person and I can find acceptable.
    Never 1 2 3 4 5 Always

Response Scale:	1	2	3	4	5
	Never	Rarely	Sometimes	Often	Always

11. I would quit a job if many conflicts occurred daily.
Never 1 2 3 4 5 Always

12. It's easier to have an outsider settle a dispute than to argue it out alone with another person.
Never 1 2 3 4 5 Always

13. I like to find what each person wants most strongly, then work for a point in the middle.
Never 1 2 3 4 5 Always

14. I hate to lose or not get my own way.
Never 1 2 3 4 5 Always

15. I like to look at lots of possibilities and options before trying to find a solution to a conflict.
Never 1 2 3 4 5 Always

16. When conflict occurs, I prefer to get out of the situation rather than work to resolve the conflict.
Never 1 2 3 4 5 Always

17. I like to take disagreements to someone who has authority and have that person make a ruling.
Never 1 2 3 4 5 Always

18. I believe resolving conflict requires that each person give up something.
Never 1 2 3 4 5 Always

19. When someone tries to get me to back down or give in during a conflict, that makes me hold my position more strongly.
Never 1 2 3 4 5 Always

20. When I especially need to have my plan accepted or when an issue is very important to me, I tell the person with whom I am in conflict.
Never 1 2 3 4 5 Always

21. I prefer to walk away from conflict if there is strong personal disagreement.
Never 1 2 3 4 5 Always

22. I prefer to have a counselor decide for two people in conflict, not just ask the two people to listen to each other.
Never 1 2 3 4 5 Always

23. I believe working out a middle-of-the-road agreement is best, even if both people are still somewhat unhappy about not getting their own way completely.
Never 1 2 3 4 5 Always

24. When I work to resolve a conflict, I work to win.
Never 1 2 3 4 5 Always

Response Scale:	1	2	3	4	5
	Never	Rarely	Sometimes	Often	Always

25. I consider the other person's preference as well as my own and work to find a solution both of us can live with.
Never 1 2 3 4 5 Always

26. I prefer to let conflicts "work themselves out."
Never 1 2 3 4 5 Always

27. I believe it is important to get the opinion of a friend when I am in conflict with someone.
Never 1 2 3 4 5 Always

28. It's okay to give up some things if the other person gives up something too.
Never 1 2 3 4 5 Always

29. I believe setting a conflict with another person is not different from competing in sports--the goal is to win.
Never 1 2 3 4 5 Always

30. I believe a conflict is really a problem, not a contest; therefore, the goal is to find a solution both people can live with, not to "beat" the other person.
Never 1 2 3 4 5 Always

Scoring: The numbers listed below refer to the statements that you have just responded to. Write down the number you circled on the scale for each statement.

1 ______	2 ______	3 ______	4 ______	5 ______
6 ______	7 ______	8 ______	9 ______	10 ______
11 ______	12 ______	13 ______	14 ______	15 ______
16 ______	17 ______	18 ______	19 ______	20 ______
21 ______	22 ______	23 ______	24 ______	25 ______
26 ______	27 ______	28 ______	29 ______	30 ______

Total Scores, each column:

A ______ Withdrawing-Avoiding	B ______ Going to a Third Person	C ______ Compromise	D ______ Win-Lose	E ______ Win-Win or Problem-Solving

List the letters and total scores from the highest down to the lowest.

Letter	Total Score	
______	______	*Highest*
______	______	
______	______	
______	______	
______	______	*Lowest*

Interpretation: The total score indicate which ways to handling conflict you use most. If two or more scores are close together (for example, compromise 30 and withdrawing-avoiding 28), you tend to use those methods about the same amount of time.

If your total score is	*You tend to use this method*
26-30	a great deal
21-25	often
16-20	sometimes
11-15	occasionally
6-10	infrequently

A. *Withdrawing-Avoiding*--handling conflict by getting away from it or ignoring it. This includes giving in quickly to avoid unpleasantness, pretending there is no conflict, moving out of the situation by quitting, breaking the relationship, or physically moving. Withdrawing may be helpful if the problem is not important to you, or if it is not a good time to discuss the disagreement. Withdrawing usually mans the other person wins.

B. *Going to a Third Person*--having a third person listen to both sides of a conflict and then help settle it. A third person can be useful if he or she helps the two people in conflict see each other's points of view. Many times, however, third persons are not fair. The success of this method depends on an unbiased third person and on whether the two people in conflict will follow what the third person recommends.

C. *Compromise*--finding a solution that allows each person to win something. Both persons may be somewhat disappointed, and yet each has the satisfaction of getting part of what he or she wanted. Most conflicts have more than two solutions, and many possibilities should be discussed before a compromise is made.

D. *Win-Lose*--holding out for your point of view or working to get the other person to give in. This is a high-risk method because you tend to win completely or lose completely. If the other person insists on trying to win totally, you have little choice but to use win-lose, unless you can get the other person to change methods.

E. *Win-Win or Problem-Solving*--looking at conflict as a problem and searching for a solution or plan that both persons feel good about. This method may end in a compromise, but usually not until after many solutions are discussed. The spotlight is on the problem, not on the personalities of the people in conflict. If personalities are the problem, then they are discussed openly, along with how each person needs to behave differently to resolve or reduce the conflict.

Source: Sandra Kammerma et al. Wellness RSVP. Menlo Park, CA: Benjamin Cummings, 1993. 51-54.

Constructive Fighting

Name: ______________________________ Date: ____________

Purpose: People who are closely involved, whether as a family, good friends, or partners, often find it difficult to resolve disagreements. One person may try to ignore a problem until it becomes very obvious and is forced into the open. Then when the issue is discussed the people involved are often dissatisfied with the outcome and the feelings they are left with. However, there are constructive methods of fighting to solve problems. This may seem too technical or mechanical, yet people find some guidelines for constructive fighting are practical, and the outcome of constructive fighting often enhances the relationship. This inventory will give you an opportunity to check your fight style.

Directions: Reach each questions carefully and respond by writing a YES or NO in the blank to the right. Respond in terms of a present relationship or a significant one from the past.

1. When your anger surfaces, do you take time to look at where it is coming from? ______
2. Whenever you argue, do you make "I" statements to explain how the other person's behavior makes you feel? ______
3. Do you say directly what change you would like to see in the current situation? ______
4. Are you sensitive to the hints your partner sends out when he/she is not happy with a situation? ______
5. Do you know what you and your partner expect of your relationship? ______
6. Do you threaten infidelity, divorce, violence, or telling others of your disagreement? ______
7. Are you dependent on your partner to fulfill many of your needs? ______
8. Are you aware of tensions that naturally occur when major lifestyle changes are made? ______
9. Do you feel that "winning" an argument is important to your self-image? ______
10. Do you keep score of who "wins" arguments? ______
11. Do you regard compromising as losing? ______
12. Are you afraid of being rejected by your partner? ______
13. Do you bring up problem areas as they arise instead of storing grudges to release all at once? ______
14. Do you belittle your partner in an attempt to control him/her? ______
15. Do you set aside a time and place where both you and your partner can discuss a problem without distractions? ______

16. Do you confine your discussions about problems to the current issue and not bring up past issues? ______

17. Are there recurring themes behind your disagreements? ______

18. If you are not sure of your partner's message, do you repeat it in your own words and ask if you understand correctly? ______

19. Do you feel you learn something from your disagreements? ______

20. Are you uneasy with the changes that may result from an argument? ______

Scoring: The questions above actually list many suggestions for constructive fighting. The correct answers are as follows:

1. YES. When you feel anger rising, it is helpful to stop to think about what is causing the anger. You need to realize that you yourself created the anger. Then ask yourself why you feel this way; it may be a result of unfair demands or expectations.

2. YES. You do not have the right to make assumptions about your partner's feelings and thoughts. Therefore, it is important to learn to begin statements with "I feel..." to let your partner know your feelings. Statements that begin "You..." tend to make assumptions and put your partner on the defensive.

3. YES. Learn to say directly what changes in the current situation you would like to see. After your partner has given his/her viewpoint, you can explore which options are fair or possible. Try to be positive in your statements, saying what you "do want" instead of focusing on the negative and what you "do not want."

4. YES. If you can understand your partner's nonverbal communication, you can ask what he/she is feeling. Your partner may want your help or support but may feel uncomfortable telling you so.

5. YES. If you have not recently discussed your expectations of your relationship, you may have conflicting ideas. Review them together to decide if any need to be change. Do not expect your partner to change just for you.

6. NO. Threats will not solve the conflict. Remember: threats are most effective if seldom used. Use them only if you feel the action is absolutely necessary and you are willing to carry it through.

7. NO. Any overdependence on your partner can cause conflict. Your partner may feel he/she is giving more than receiving. Take a look at your needs and reevaluate how to meet them.

8. YES. Many lifestyle changes naturally result in more tension and stress. Be aware of those situations and avoid blaming your partner for the stress.

9. NO. If you feel you must "win" an argument to keep your self-image, think about where your real happiness in the relationship comes from. Solving the problem that caused the conflict is the most important factor.

10. NO. Do not keep score of who "wins." Again the real issue is that the conflict is resolved. Keeping score tends to make people want to "get even." Stable relationships involve cooperation.

11. NO. Again, the real issue is that the conflict is resolved. A compromise is usually best since there is no "loser" whose feelings are hurt.

12. NO. If communication is open in your relationship, your partner will not reject you because you do not always agree. In fact, couples often find conflict resolution serves to strengthen a relationship.

13. YES. It is easier to find a compromise for problem issues if they are discussed and resolved one at a time as they arise. If one partner holds grudges for a period of time, it may cause conflicts in other areas.

14. NO Attempting to belittle your partner is likely to put him/her on the defensive. In addition, the real concern should be reaching a compromise together.

15. YES. When a conflict needs to be resolved, one partner may want to make an appointment with the other. Discussion should not take place while either partner is tired, rushed, or under the influence of alcohol or drugs. Both partners need to be able to devote their full attention to the issue. If one person has an important presentation to make or paper to write, the discussion may need to be delayed for a reasonable length of time.

16. YES. Discussions should be limited to the current problem since it is better to deal with one issue at at time. If an unresolved issue is brought up, agree to discuss it at a later time.

17. NO. If the same arguments or variations on the same theme keep recurring, perhaps you need to look at your process for conflict resolution. Ask yourself if any positive changes have been made since the last time you discussed the issue.

18. YES. This is a basic rule of good communication. Restate what you heard your partner say but in your own words. This helps to clear up misunderstandings before they become problems.

19. YES. When fighting is constructive, both partners will learn something about themselves and their partner. This new information can then be applied to similar situations that arise in the future. Thus, no conflict would result.

20. NO. Both partners should feel 20. NO. Both partners should feel fairly comfortable with the changes agreed upon, although feel completely comfortable if they are changing habits developed over several years. Both partners need encouragement and positive strokes when making changes.

Now that you have evaluated your fight style, try to practice these suggestions the next time you feel angry or disagree with someone. Remember, these basic guidelines can be applied to disagreements with anyone--partner, mate, co-worker, or family member. However, if you cannot solve the problem, seek professional help. Friends and family may be able to help some, but a potentially long-term relationship is too important to trust to well-meaning friends. Seek professional help together. Once you resolve the conflict, put the problem behind you and have some fun!

Source: Robert F. Valois and Sandra Kammerman. Your Sexuality: A Self Assessment, 2nd Ed. New York: McGraw Hill, 1992. 113-116.

Test Your Sleep I.Q.

The following true or false statements test what you know about sleep. Be sure to read the correct answers and explanations.

True False 1. Sleep is a time when your body and brain shut down for rest and relaxation.

True False 2. If you regularly doze off unintentionally during the day, you may need more than just a good night's sleep.

True False 3. If you snore loudly and persistently at night and are sleepy during the day, you may have a sleep disorder.

True False 4. Opening the car window or turning the radio up will keep the drowsy driver awake.

True False 5. Narcolepsy is a sleep disorder marked by "sleep attacks."

True False 6. The primary cause of insomnia is worry.

True False 7. One cause of not getting enough sleep is restless legs syndrome.

True False 8. The body has a natural ability to adjust to different sleep schedules such as working different shifts or traveling through multiple time zones quickly.

True False 9. People need less sleep as they grow older.

True False 10. More people doze off at the wheel of a car in the early morning or midafternoon than in the evening.

Scoring

1. False.
Although it is a time when your body rests and restores its energy levels, sleep is an active state that affects both your physical and mental well-being. Adequate restful sleep, like diet and exercise, is critical to good health. Insufficient restful sleep can result in mental and physical health problems and possibly premature death.

2. True.
Many people doze off unintentionally during the day despite getting their usual night of sleep. This could be a sign of a sleep disorder. Approximately 40 million Americans suffer from sleep disorders, including sleep apnea, insomnia, narcolepsy, and restless legs syndrome. An untreated sleep disorder can reduce your daytime productivity, increase your risk of accidents, and put you at risk for illness and even early death.

3. True.
Persistent loud snoring at night and daytime sleepiness are the main symptoms of a common and serious sleep disorder, sleep apnea. Another symptom is frequent long pauses in breathing during sleep, followed by choking and gasping for breath. People with sleep apnea don't get enough restful sleep, and their daytime performance is often seriously affected. Sleep apnea may also lead to hypertension, heart disease,

heart attack, and stroke. However, it can be treated, and the sleep apnea patient can live a normal life.

4. False.
Opening the car window or turning the radio up may arouse a drowsy driver briefly, but this won't keep that person alert behind the wheel. Even mild drowsiness is enough to reduce concentration and reaction time. The sleep-deprived driver may nod off for a couple of seconds at a time without even knowing it--enough time to kill himself or someone else. It has been estimated that drowsy driving may account for an average of 56,000 reported accidents each year--claiming over 1,500 lives.

5. True.
People with narcolepsy fall asleep uncontrollably --at any time of the day, in all types of situations --regardless of the amount or quality of sleep they've had the night before. Narcolepsy is characterized by these "sleep attacks," as well as by daytime sleepiness, episodes of muscle weakness or paralysis, and disrupted nighttime sleep. Although there is no known cure, medications and behavioral treatments can control symptoms, and people with narcolepsy can live normal lives.

6. False.
Insomnia has many different causes, including physical and mental conditions and stress. Insomnia is the perception that you don't get enough sleep because you can't fall asleep or stay asleep or get back to sleep once you've awakened during the night. It affects people of all ages, usually for just an occasional night or two, but sometimes for weeks, months, or even years. Because insomnia can become a chronic problem, it is important to get it diagnosed and treated if it persists for more than a month.

7. True.
Restless legs syndrome (RLS) is a medical condition distinguished by tingling sensations in the legs--and sometimes the arms--while sitting or lying still, especially at bedtime. The person with RLS needs to constantly stretch or move the legs to try to relieve these uncomfortable or painful symptoms. As a result, he or she has difficulty falling asleep or staying asleep and usually feels extremely sleepy and unable to function fully during the day. Good sleep habits and medication can help the person with RLS.

8. False.
The human body's biological clock programs each person to feel sleepy during the nighttime hours and to be active during the daylight hours. So people who work the night shift and try to sleep during the day are constantly fighting their biological clocks. This puts them at risk of error and accident at work and of disturbed sleep. The same is true for people who travel through multiple time zones quickly; they get "jet lag" because they cannot maintain a regular sleep-wake schedule. Sleeping during the day in a dark, quiet bedroom and getting exposure to sufficient bright light at the right time can help improve daytime alertness.

9. False.
As we get older, we don't need less sleep, but we often get less sleep. That's because our ability to sleep for long periods of time and to get into the deep restful stages of sleep decreases with age. Older people have more fragile sleep and are more easily disturbed by light, noise, and pain. They also may have medical conditions that contribute to sleep problems. Going to bed at the same time every night and getting up at the same time every morning, getting exposure to natural outdoor light during the day, and sleeping in a cool, dark, quiet place at night may help.

10. True. Our bodies are programmed by our biological clock to experience two natural periods of

sleepiness during the 24-hour day, regardless of the amount of sleep we've had in the previous 24 hours. The primary period is between about midnight and 7:00 a.m. A second period of less intense sleepiness is in the midafternoon, between about 1:00 and 3:00. This means that we are more at risk of falling asleep at the wheel at these times than in the evening--especially if we haven't been getting enough sleep.

HOW MANY ANSWERS DID YOU GET CORRECT?

9-10 Correct
Congratulation! You know a lot about sleep. Share this information with your family and friends

7-8 Correct
Very Good.

Fewer Than 7 Correct
Go over the answers and try to learn more about sleep.

Source: U.S. Department of Health and Human Services, Public Institute Service, National Institutes of Health, National Heart, Lung and Blood Institute

The Family Stress Test: How Stressed is Your Family?

Directions

Take this quiz to help you evaluate your family's stress level. Score:

0 if the statement is never true for your family
1 if the statement is rarely true
2 if the statement is sometimes true
3 if the statement is always true

PART A:

_____ 1. We often talk about our feelings.
_____ 2. I know what is important to my kids.
_____ 3. (For single parents)I'm comfortable being single.
_____ 4. We have enough money for important things.
_____ 5. Work is important, but family is our top priority.
_____ 6. (For couples)Our relationship is strong.
_____ 7. (For couples)We both feel good about our roles as parents.
_____ 8. (For single parents)The kids like my choice of dates.
_____ 9. Tension in our house is rare.
_____ 10. The kids are doing well in school.
_____ 11. Everyone in the family has a job and does it without being nagged.
_____ 12. We eat together every day.
_____ 13. Vacations together turn out well.

TOTAL SCORE PART A: _____

PART B:

_____ 1. It seems we argue a lot.
_____ 2. We don't listen enough.
_____ 3. (For single parents)Being single has been very hard for me.
_____ 4. We have conflicts about how much to spend and on what..
_____ 5. It's impossible to get the kids to do anything around here.
_____ 6. (For couples)We argue about who should do what with the kids.
_____ 7. (For couples)Sometimes marriage is disappointing.
_____ 8. (For single parents)My kids are upset when I date.
_____ 9. Too much work is getting to me.
_____ 10. It seems as if someone is always mad at someone else.
_____ 11. There is never enough time.
_____ 12. The kids get upset that we argue.
_____ 13. I have been called in to school to discuss my child's behavior.

TOTAL SCORE PART B: _____

Scoring

For Part A scores of 33 and above and/or Part B scores of 17 or less:
Congratulations! Your family has good skills and attitudes which help you handle life's stresses. This makes your home life rich and satisfying.

For Part A scores of 25-32 and/or Part B scores of 18-24:
You have a strong start. Try practicing your good skills and positive attitudes more, to create even more harmony at home

For Part A scores of 18-24 and/or Part B scores of 25-32:
You're probably under many stresses. Look carefully at these questions and think about ways to improve your score. Remember it is not a sign of weakness to ask for help.

For Part A scores of 17 or less and/or Part B scores of 33 and above:
Taking action now is very important for your family's health and happiness. Reach out to friends, family or professional help for a great boost when times are tough.

Source: FOCUS ON HEALTH Newsletter, Spring 1999, http://jeeves.niehs.nih.gov/odhsb/focus/spring99/stress.html

HOW YOU DEAL WITH YOUR STRESS

Listed below are things people may do when they experience stress.

Think back over the recent past. Think about how you coped with any problems or stressful situations that you faced in the recent past.

Put a check in Column 1 to show how often you did each thing when you experienced stress.
Put a check in Column 2 to show whether or not the action helped to reduce your stress.
If you checked NEVER in Column 1, you do not need to answer Column 2 for that item.

	Column 1			Column 2		
In the ***recent past***, when you felt stress, how often did you...				Did it help to ***reduce your stress?***		
	A Lot	Sometimes	Never	A Lot	A Little	No
1. think about the good things in your life?						
2. try to figure out what upset you about the problem?						
3. use relaxation skills?						
4. try to see the good side of the situation?						
5. exercise more?						
6. smoke cigarettes?						
7. think about how you would handle the situation?						
8. try to get more information about the situation?						
9. make a plan of action and follow it?						
10. have a drink (such as beer or wine)?						
11. accept the situation if nothing could be done to change it?						

12. do other things for awhile to get your mind off the situation?						
13. get high?						
14. talk about your feelings with your family?						
15. take your anger out on other people?						
16. learn new skills to help you deal with the situation?						
17. ask others for help if you needed it?						
18. take the blame for a problem that wasn't your fault?						
19. keep your feelings to yourself?						
20. think. about some different ways to handle the situation?						
21. talk about your feelings with your friends?						

Source: Instrument adapted from How You Deal with Your Stress, in *Program Evaluation Handbook: Stress Management*, 1988, Los Angeles, CA: IOX Assessment Associates, pp. 44-48

How You Deal with Your Stress
Scoring and Analysis

This behavior measure examine the frequency with which participants have used a variety of stress management techniques during the recent past. After describing frequency of use, participants indicate how helpful each technique was in reducing stress. Both positive and negative techniques for managing stress are included on the measure.

Column 1: Frequency

Items 6, 10, 13, 15, 18, and 19 are commonly considered some of the negative ways for handling stress. For purposes of scoring, they will be labeled "negative items."

The remaining items are positive coping techniques. They will be labeled "positive items."

Total Score for Negative Items Marked A LOT or SOMETIMES
1. Count the number of negative items that are marked either A LOT or SOMETIMES. (Ignore any blank or NEVER responses.)
2. Divide this total by the number of program participants.

EXAMPLE. Imagine that there are 10 program participants. First, count all the times that these individuals marked either A LOT or SOMETIMES on the negative items (6, 10, 13, 15, 18, and 19). Let's assume the total number of times was 32. Then, divide 32 by 10 participants to get an average score of 3.2. Scores can range from 0-6 with low numbers indicating a group of participants who use few negative coping techniques and high numbers indicating the use of many negative techniques.

Subtotal Score for Negative Items Marked A LOT or SOMETIMES
1. Count only the number of negative items (6, 10, 13, 15, 18, and 19) that are marked A LOT.
2. Divide this total by the number of times the negative items were marked A LOT or SOMETIMES. Multiply this number times 100 to obtain a percentage.

EXAMPLE. For the same 10 individuals used in the example above, count the number of times they marked A LOT on the negative items. Let's assume the total was 11. Then, divide by the total number of times the 10 individuals marked either A LOT or SOMETIMES on the negative items. This number was already determined to be 32 in the previous example. And, divide 11 by 32 to find out, of the negative strategies used, what percent are used A LOT, find out, of the negative strategies used, what percent are used A LOT. In this case, 11/32 is about 34%. Thus, of negative strategies used, 34% are used often, and 66 % are used sometimes.

Scoring for Positive Items Marked A LOT or SOMETIMES

Items measuring frequency of use of positive techniques for handling stress can be scored in the same manner as the negative items. However, in this case, because of the larger number of positive items on the instrument, the possible range of scores is from 0-15 with low scores indicating the use of few positive coping strategies and high numbers indicating the use of many positive strategies. The determination of percentages for the SOMETIMES and A LOT columns can also be done with the positive strategies. It would be desirable to see a higher percentage of A LOTs being reported for the use of positive coping strategies.

Note: When dealing with the scoring of positive stress management techniques, you should not be overly concerned about group scores that do not extend into the upper end of the range. It seems unlikely that even the most skilled positive stress management participants would use all the positive coping strategies listed. Rather, individual participants may find several positive strategies that work well for them.

Column 2: Did it help to reduce your stress?

Information from Column 2 indicates participants' perceptions regarding the effectiveness of the positive techniques that they use to cope with stress. is column can be scored by focusing on the positive items (see paragraph one under Column 1: Frequency).

Scoring:

1. Count the number of positive items marked A LOT or A LITTLE.
2. Divide that total by the total number of positive items marked A LOT or SOMETIMES in Column 1. (Be sure not to include any responses marked NEVER in Column 1.)
3. Multiply by 100 to obtain a percentage.
4. Repeat steps 1 - 3 with positive items marked NO.

The percentages give you an indication of the your perception of the effectiveness of the positive stress management techniques being used.

EXAMPLE- For the same 10 individuals used in the examples above, count the number of positive items (any item that is not 6, 10, 13, 15, 18, and 19) that they marked A LOT or A LITTLE. Let's assume that this total was 95. Now, count the number of positive items marked A LOT or SOMETIMES in Column 1; let's divide the Column 21 total by the Column I total. In this case 95/140 is about .68 or 68%. Thus, 68% the participants felt that they were helped to some degree by the positive coping strategies they used. The percentage of positive items marked NO could be obtained using the same method.

Your Ideas About Decisions

Directions

The sentences below are about making decisions. For each sentence, place a check to show how much you agree or disagree with the sentence.

Strongly Agree = SA
Agree = A
Not Sure = NS
Disagree = D
Strongly Disagree = SD

SA	A	NS	D	SD	
					1. It is worth the time it takes to make decisions carefully.
					2. People should go with their first ideas when making decisions.
					3. People are happier with their decisions when they take the time to make them carefully.
					4. Spending a lot of time to make careful decisions is too difficult.
					5. Making careful decisions takes too much time.
					6. When making decisions, people should do what they feel, not what they think.
					7. People make equally good decisions no matter how they arrive at them.
					8. People who make quick decisions are usually disappointed with them later.
					9. People should take time to make decisions carefully.
					10. It is easy to make decisions carefully.

Scoring

Point values are assigned to responses as follows:

Item No.	Strongly Agree	Agree	Not Sure	Disagree	Strongly Disagree
1	5	4	3	2	1
2	1	2	3	4	5
3	5	3	3	2	1
4	1	2	3	4	5
5	1	2	3	4	5
6	1	2	3	4	5
7	1	2	3	4	5
8	5	4	3	2	1
9	5	4	3	2	1
10	5	4	3	2	1

This inventory can be scored by adding the point values of the responses from all participants and dividing this total by the number of responses (10). Blank items should not be counted in the number of responses. The maximum attainable score of 5 points indicates a strong belief in the utility of making decisions carefully. A minimum score of 1 indicates a weak belief in the utility of making decisions carefully.

Source: Adapted from CDC, *Program Evaluation Handbook: Stress Management*, 1988, IOX Assessment Associates.

Rating the Evening News

I - Aggressive Acts

Name: ______________________________ Date: __________

1. Which network news program did you watch? (circle one)
   ABC CBS NBC Other ____________________

2. What time was the broadcast? From ________ until _________

3. Who was the anchor reading the news? ____________________

4. How many separate stories or news items were presented during the broadcast? ______________

5. How many separate stories focused on some kind of aggressive act or aggressive behavior? ______________

6. Briefly describe each of the news stories that focused on aggression. In which position did each story appear during the newscast (i.e., was it the first story? the fifth story? the last story?)

Description	Position
______________________________	______________
______________________________	______________
______________________________	______________
______________________________	______________
______________________________	______________
______________________________	______________
______________________________	______________
______________________________	______________
______________________________	______________
______________________________	______________

7. Divide the number of stories that focused on aggression by the total number of stories presented during the broadcast.

Number of stories on aggression ______ divided by

Total number of stories ____________ = ______

II - Prosocial Acts

1. Which network news program did you watch? (circle one)
   ABC CBS NBC Other ____________________

2. What time was the broadcast? From ________ until _________

3. Who was the anchor reading the news? ________________________

4. How many separate stories or news items were presented during the broadcast? __________________

5. How many separate stories focused on some kind of prosocial act or prosocial behavior (i.e., someone who gave help or someone who acted unselfishly)? __________________

6. Briefly describe each of the news stories that focused on prosocial behavior. In which position did each story appear during the newscast (i.e., was it the first story? the fifth story? the last story?)

Description	Position
____	___________________
____	___________________
____	___________________
____	___________________
____	___________________
____	___________________
____	___________________
____	___________________
____	___________________
____	___________________

7. Divide the number of stories that focused on aggression by the total number of stories presented ruing the broadcast.

Number of stories on aggression _______ divided by

Total number of stories _______________ = ________

Coercive Sex Questionnaire

Name: ______________________________ Date: ____________

Sexual coercion places both men and women in "victim" roles, although women are victimized more often.

The development of effective strategies to deal with the problem of coercive sex requires changing the traditional gender role socialization that makes females vulnerable to sexual abuse and pushes males into the "victimizer" role. Decisions to make such changes are usually based upon our values and attitudes toward the use of power and influence.

Purpose: The exercise that follows is designed to assist you in clarifying your choices about ways to deal the problem of coercive sex.

Directions: Write in the feelings and behaviors you would most likely experience or engage in for each of the first eight questions. In question 9, check the appropriate box to identify your choice.

1. If you were witnessing a rape of a stranger in a public place (e.g., bus depot)...

   a) How would you feel?

   b) What would you do?

2. If your spouse were the victim of a forcible rape...

   a) How would you feel?

   b) What would you do?

3. If you learned that a child in your neighborhood was being subjected to an incestuous relationship with his or her parent...

   a) How would you feel?

   b) What would you do?

4. If you learned that two of your children (e.g., son and daughter) were involved in brother-sister incest...

   a) How would you feel?

   b) What would you do?

5. If you learned that your spouse was asked to participate in sexual activity with his or her boss in order to keep a job or get a promotion...

   a) How would you feel?

   b) What would you do?

6. If you were applying for a position of employment that you wanted very badly and the prospective employer made it clear that hiring depended on your sexual "availability" and requested a "sample" as a sign of "good faith"...

a) How would you feel?

b) What would you do?

7. If you were constantly stared at, touched, and visually and verbally "raped" and generally taken advantage of at work...

a) How would you feel?

b) What would you do?

8. If you were invited to a private showing of sexually explicit movies at a neighbor's home and realized that the films you were viewing were of young children engaged in sexual activity...

a) How would you feel?

b) What would you do?

9. If a referendum appeared on the ballot in your state to require mandatory sentence for coercive sexual behavior, how would you vote on the following? Place a check mark in the appropriate space.

	Sentence		
	Long Term	Short Term	None
Coercive Sex	______	______	______
Forcible rape	______	______	______
Statutory rape	______	______	______
Parent-child incest	______	______	______
Sibling incest	______	______	______
Sexual harassment at work	______	______	______

Scoring: Responses to this inventory would be very specific to each individual. Taking a closer look at these issues and discussing them with significant others may help you clarify your feelings in regard to coercive sex.

Source: Robert F. Valois and Sandra Kammerman. Your Sexuality: A Self-Assessment, 2nd Ed. New York, McGraw-Hill, 1992. 113-116

Household Poison Safety Checklist

Directions

Indicate “Yes” or “No” in response to each statement.

Medicine Safety

Yes No When using child-resistant packaging, I read the instructions to make it easier to open the packaging.

Yes No When using child-resistant packaging, I am sure to resecure the closure tightly.

Yes No When using child-resistant packaging, I never transfer the contents to other containers.

Yes No I do not leave loose pills anywhere.

Yes No I always leave the light on when giving or taking medicines.

Yes No I avoid taking medicines in front of children, since youngsters tend to imitate grown-ups.

Yes No I refer to medicine as "medicine" - not "candy."

Yes No I clean out the medicine cabinet periodically, and safely dispose of unneeded medicines when the illness for which they were prescribed is over. Pour contents down drain or toilet, and rinse container before discarding.

Yes No I always read the label and follow instructions when taking medicines. If any questions arise, I consult my physician.

Yes No I never mix medicines and alcohol, and never take more than the prescribed amount of medicine.

Yes No I never "borrow" a friend's medicine or take old medicines.

Yes No I tell my doctor what other medicines I am taking so you can avoid adverse drug interactions.

Yes No I inspect the outer packaging on over-the-counter medicines to check for tampering.

Yes No I don't use any medicine from a package that shows cuts, slices, tears, or other imperfections.

Yes No I read the label and look at the medicine every time I take a dose.

Chemical Safety

Yes No I keep medicines and household chemical products (even those with safety caps) out of sight whenever children are in the house.

Yes No I use locks or child- resistant latches to secure storage areas for medicines and household products whenever children are in the house.

Yes No I never use cups or soft-drink bottles to hold paint thinner, turpentine, gasoline, or other household chemicals.

Yes No I store all medicines separately from household products, and store all household chemical products away from food.

Yes No I keep all household chemical product items in their original containers.

Yes No I leave the original labels on all products.

Yes No I do not put decorative lamps and candles that contain lamp oil where children can reach them.

Pesticide Safety

Yes No I always store pesticides away from children's reach, in a locked cabinet or garden shed.

Yes	No	I read pesticide labels first and follow the directions to the letter, including all precautions and restrictions.
Yes	No	Before applying pesticides (indoors and outdoors), I remove children and their toys from the area and keep them away until it is dry or as recommended by the label.
Yes	No	I never leave pesticides unattended when I am using them - not even for a few minutes.
Yes	No	I never transfer pesticides to other containers.
Yes	No	I use child-resistant packaging for pesticides properly by closing the container tightly after use.
Yes	No	When using pesticides, I alert others to the potential hazard, especially grandparents and caregivers.

Scoring

Every "Yes" response suggests that you are taking measures to protect your family and yourself from household poisoning.

Every "No" response describes a situation in which the potential for household poisoning from medicine or pesticides exists.

Source: Adapted from Poison Prevention Week EDITOR'S FACT SHEET CPSC Document 386,
The U.S. Consumer Product Safety Commission

Can Your Kitchen Pass the Food Safety Test?

Directions

Choose the answer that best describes the practice in your household, whether or not you are the primary food handler.

1. The temperature of the refrigerator in my home is:
   a. 50 degrees Fahrenheit (10 degrees Celsius).
   b. 41 F (5 C).
   c. I don't know; I've never measured it.

2. The last time we had leftover cooked stew or other food with meat, chicken or fish, the food was:
   a. cooled to room temperature, then put in the refrigerator.
   b. put in the refrigerator immediately after the food was served.
   c. left at room temperature overnight or longer.

3. The last time the kitchen sink drain, disposal and connecting pipe in my home were sanitized was:
   a. last night.
   b. several weeks ago.
   c. can't remember.

4. If a cutting board is used in my home to cut raw meat, poultry or fish and it is going to be used to chop another food, the board is:
   a. reused as is.
   b. wiped with a damp cloth.
   c. washed with soap and hot water.
   d. washed with soap and hot water and then sanitized.

5. The last time we had hamburgers in my home, I ate mine:
   a. rare.
   b. medium.
   c. well-done.

6. The last time there was cookie dough in my home, the dough was:
   a. ate with raw eggs, and I sampled some of it.
   b. tore-bought, and I sampled some of it.
   c. not sampled until baked.

7. I clean my kitchen counters and other surfaces that come in contact with food with:
   a. water.
   b. hot water and soap.
   c. hot water and soap, then bleach solution.
   d. hot water and soap, then commercial sanitizing agent.

8. When dishes are washed in my home, they are:
   a. cleaned by an automatic dishwasher and then air-dried.
   b. left to soak in the sink for several hours and then washed with soap in the same water.
   c. washed right away with hot water and soap in the sink and then air-dried.
   d. washed right away with hot water and soap in the sink and immediately towel-dried.

9. The last time I handled raw meat, poultry or fish, I cleaned my hands afterwards by:
   a. wiping them on a towel.
   b. rinsing them under hot, cold or warm tap water.
   c. washing with soap and warm water.

10. Meat, poultry and fish products are defrosted in my home by:
    a. setting them on the counter .
    b. placing them in the refrigerator.
    c. microwaving.

11. When I buy fresh seafood, I:
    a. buy only fish that's refrigerated or well iced.
    b. take it home immediately and put it in the refrigerator.
    c. sometimes buy it straight out of a local fisher's creel.

12. I realize people, including myself, should be especially careful about not eating raw seafood, if they have:
    a. diabetes
    b. HIV infection
    c. cancer
    d. liver disease

Scoring and Answers

1. Refrigerators should stay at 41 F (5 C) or less, so if you chose answer B, give yourself two points.

2. Answer B is the best practice; give yourself two points if you picked it.
Hot foods should be refrigerated as soon as possible within two hours after cooking. But don't keep the food if it's been standing out for more than two hours.

3. If answer A best describes your household's practice, give yourself two points. Give yourself one point if you chose B.
The kitchen sink drain, disposal and connecting pipe are often overlooked, but they should be sanitized periodically by pouring down the sink a solution of 1 teaspoon (5 milliliters) of chlorine bleach in 1 quart (about 1 liter) of water or a solution of commercial kitchen cleaning agent made according to product directions.

4. If answer D best describes your household's practice, give yourself two points.
If you picked A, you're violating an important food safety rule: Never allow raw meat, poultry and fish to come in contact with other foods. Answer B isn't good, either. Improper washing, such as with a damp cloth, will not remove bacteria.

5. Give yourself two points if you picked answer C.

6. If you answered A, you may be putting yourself at risk for infection with Salmonella enteritidis, a bacterium that can be in shell eggs.
Cooking the egg or egg-containing food product to an internal temperature of at least 145 F (63 C) kills the bacteria. So answer C--eating the baked product--will earn you two points.
You'll get two points for answer B, also. Foods containing raw eggs, such as homemade ice cream, cake batter, mayonnaise, and eggnog, carry a Salmonella risk, but their commercial counterparts don't.

7. Answers C or D will earn you two points each; answer B, one point.
Bleach and commercial kitchen cleaning agents are the best sanitizers--provided they're diluted according to product directions.

8. Answers A and C are worth two points each.
There are potential problems with B and D. When you let dishes sit in water for a long time, it "creates a soup," FDA's Buchanan said. When washing dishes by hand, he said, it's best to wash them all within two hours.

9. The only correct practice is answer C. Give yourself two points if you picked it.
Wash hands with warm water and soap for at least 20 seconds before and after handling food, especially raw meat, poultry and fish. If you have an infection or cut on your hands, wear rubber or plastic gloves.

10. Give yourself two points if you picked B or C.
Food safety experts recommend thawing foods in the refrigerator or the microwave oven or putting the package in a water-tight plastic bag submerged in cold water and changing the water every 30 minutes.

11. A and B are correct. Give yourself two points for either.
When buying fresh seafood, buy only from reputable dealers who keep their products refrigerated or properly iced.

12. If you are under treatment for any of these diseases, as well as several others, you should avoid raw seafood. Give yourself two points for knowing one or more of the risky conditions.
Rating Your Home's Food Practices

24 points: Feel confident about the safety of foods served in your home.

12 to 23 points: Reexamine food safety practices in your home. Some key rules are being violated.

11 points or below: Take steps immediately to correct food handling, storage and cooking techniques used in your home. Current practices are putting you and other members of your household in danger of food-borne illness.

Source: "Can Your Kitchen Pass the Food Safety Test?" by Paula Kurtzweil, FDA Consumer. October 1998.

Home Safety Checklist

Directions

Use this checklist to spot possible safety problems which may be present in your home. Check YES or NO to answer each question.

YES ___ NO ___ 1. Are lamp, extension, and telephone cords placed out of the flow of traffic?

RECOMMENDATION: Arrange furniture so that outlets are available for lamps and appliances without the use of extension cords. If you must use an extension cord, place it on the floor against a wall where people can not trip over it.

YES ___ No ___ 2. Are cords out from beneath furniture and rugs or carpeting?

RECOMMENDATION: Remove cords from under furniture or carpeting. Replace damaged or frayed cords.

YES ___ NO ___ 3. Are cords attached to the walls, baseboards, etc., with nails or staples?

RECOMMENDATION: Remove nails, staples, etc. Check wiring for damage. Use tape to attach cords to walls or floors.

YES ___ NO ___ 4. Are electrical cords in good condition, not frayed or cracked?

RECOMMENDATION: Replace frayed or cracked cords.

YES ___ NO ___ 5. Do extension cords carry more than their proper load, as indicated by the ratings labeled on the cord and the appliance?

RECOMMENDATION: Standard 18 gauge extension cords can carry 1250 watts. If the rating on the cord is exceeded because of the power requirements of one or more appliances being used on the cord, change the cord to a higher rated one or unplug some appliances. If an extension cord is needed, use one having a sufficient amp or wattage rating.

YES ___ NO ___ 6. Are all small rugs and runners slip-resistant?

RECOMMENDATION: Remove rugs and runners that tend to slide. Apply double-faced adhesive carpet tape or rubber matting to the backs of rugs and runners. Purchase rugs with slip-resistant backing. Check rugs and mats periodically to see if backing needs to be replaced. Place rubber matting under rugs. (Rubber matting that can be cut to size is available.) Purchase new rugs with slip-resistant backing.

YES ___ NO ___ 7. Are emergency numbers posted on or near the telephone?

RECOMMENDATION: In case of emergency, telephone numbers for the Police, Fire Department, and local Poison Control Center, along with a neighbor's number, should be readily available. Write the numbers in large print and tape them to the phone, or place them near the phone where they can be seen easily.

YES ___ NO ___ 8. Do you have access to a telephone if you fall (or experience some other emergency which prevents you from standing and reaching a wall phone)?

RECOMMENDATION: Have at least one telephone located where it would be accessible in the event of an accident which leaves you unable to stand.

YES ___ NO___ 9. Are smoke detectors properly located?

RECOMMENDATION: At least one smoke detector should be placed on every floor of your home. Read the instructions that come with the smoke detector for advice on the best place to install it. Make sure detectors are placed near bedrooms, either on the ceiling or 6-12 inches below the ceiling on the wall. Locate smoke detectors away from air vents.

YES ___ NO ___ 10. Do you have properly working smoke detectors?

RECOMMENDATION: Many home fire injuries and deaths are caused by smoke and toxic gases, rather than the fire itself. Smoke detectors provide an early warning and can wake you in the event of a fire. Purchase a smoke detector if you do not have one. Check and replace batteries and bulbs according to the manufacturer's instructions. Vacuum the grillwork of your smoke detector. Replace any smoke detectors which can not be repaired.

YES ___ NO ___ 11. Are any outlets and switches unusually warm or hot to the touch?

RECOMMENDATION: Unusually warm or hot outlets or switches may indicate that an unsafe wiring condition exists. Unplug cords from outlets and do not use the switches. Have an electrician check the wiring as soon as possible.

YES ___ NO ___ 12. Do all outlets and switches have cover plates, so that no wiring is exposed?

RECOMMENDATION: Exposed wiring presents a shock hazard. Add a cover plate.

YES ___ NO ___ 13. Are light bulbs the appropriate size and type for the lamp or fixture?

RECOMMENDATION: A bulb of too high wattage or the wrong type may lead to fire through overheating. Ceiling fixtures, recessed lights, and "hooded" lamps will trap heat. Replace with a bulb of the correct type and wattage.

YES ___ NO ___ 14. Are heaters which come with a 3-prong plug being used in a 3-hole outlet or with a properly attached adapter?

RECOMMENDATION: The grounding feature provided by a 3-hole receptacle or an adapter for a 2-hole receptacle is a safety feature designed to lessen the risk of shock.

YES ___ NO ___ 15. Are small stoves and heaters placed where they can not be knocked over, and away from furnishings and flammable materials, such as curtains or rugs?

RECOMMENDATION: Heaters can cause fires or serious burns if they cause you to trip or if they are knocked over. Relocate heaters away from passageways and flammable materials such as curtains, rugs, furniture, etc.

YES ___ NO ___ 16. If your home has space heating equipment, such as a kerosene heater, a gas heater or an LP gas heater, do you understand the installation and operating instructions thoroughly?

RECOMMENDATION: Unvented heaters should be used with room doors open or window slightly open to provide ventilation. The correct fuel, as recommended by the manufacturer, should always be used. Vented heaters should have proper venting, and the venting system should be checked frequently.

YES ___ NO ___ 17. Is woodburning equipment installed properly?

RECOMMENDATION: Woodburning stoves should be installed by a qualified person according to local building codes.

YES ___ NO ___ 18. Do you have an emergency exit plan and an alternate emergency exit plan in case of a fire?

RECOMMENDATION: Develop an emergency exit plan. Choose a meeting place outside your home so you can be sure that everyone is capable of escape quickly and safely. Practice the plan from time to time to make sure everyone is capable of escape quickly and safely. Remember periodically to re-check your home.

YES ___ NO ___ 19. Are towels, curtains, and other things that might catch fire located away from the range?

RECOMMENDATION: Store flammable and combustible items away from range and oven.

YES ___ NO ___ 20. Do you wear clothing with short or close-fitting sleeves while you are cooking?

RECOMMENDATION: Roll back long, loose sleeves or fasten them with pins or elastic bands while you are cooking.

YES ___ NO ___ 21. Are kitchen ventilation systems or range exhausts functioning properly and are they in use while you are cooking?

RECOMMENDATION: Indoor air pollutants may accumulate to unhealthful levels in a kitchen where gas or kerosene-fire appliances are in use. Use ventilation systems or open windows to clear air of vapors and smoke.

YES ___ NO ___ 22. Are all extension cords and appliance cords located away from the sink or range areas?

RECOMMENDATION: Electrical appliances and power cords can cause shock or electrocution if they come in contact with water. Cords can also be damaged by excess heat. Move cords and appliances away from sink areas and hot surfaces. Move appliances closer to wall outlets or to different outlets so you won't need extension cords.

YES ___ NO ___ 23. Does good, even lighting exist over the stove, sink, and countertop work areas, especially where food is sliced or cut?

RECOMMENDATION: Low lighting and glare can contribute to burns or cuts. Improve lighting.

YES ___ NO ___ 24. Do you have a step stool which is stable and in good repair?

RECOMMENDATION: If you don't have a step stool, consider buying one. Choose one with a handrail that you can hold onto while standing on the top step. Before climbing on any step stool, make sure it is fully opened and stable.

YES ___ NO ___ 25. Are chimneys clear from accumulations of leaves, and other debris that can clog them?

RECOMMENDATION: A clogged chimney can cause a poorly-burning fire to result in poisonous fumes and smoke coming back into the house. Do not use the chimney until the blockage has been removed. Have the chimney checked and cleaned by a registered or licensed professional.

YES ___ NO ___ 26. Are hallways, passageways between rooms, and other heavy traffic areas well lit?

RECOMMENDATION: Shadowed or dark areas can hide tripping hazards. Install night lights.

YES ___ NO ___ 27. Are exits and passageways kept clear?

RECOMMENDATION: Furniture, boxes, or other items could be an obstruction or tripping hazard, especially in the event of an emergency or fire. Rearrange furniture to open passageways and walkways. Remove boxes and clutter.

YES ___ NO ___ 28. Are bathtubs and showers equipped with non-skid mats, abrasive strips, or surfaces that are not slippery?

RECOMMENDATION: Wet soapy tile or porcelain surfaces are especially slippery and may contribute to falls. Apply textured strips or appliques on the floors of tubs and showers. Use non-skid mats in the tub and shower, and on the bathroom floor.

YES ___ NO ___ 29. Is the temperature 120 degrees or lower?

RECOMMENDATION: Water temperature above 120 degrees can cause tap water scalds. Lower the setting on your hot water heater to "Low" or 120 degrees.

YES ___ NO ___ 30. Is a light switch located near the entrance to the bathroom?

RECOMMENDATIONS: A light switch near the door will prevent you from walking through a dark area. Install a night light. Inexpensive lights that plug into outlets are available.

YES ___ NO ___ 31. Are small electrical appliances such as hair dryers, shavers, curling irons, etc., unplugged when not in use?

RECOMMENDATION: Even an appliance that is not turned on, such as a hairdryer, can be potentially hazardous if it is left plugged in. If it falls into water in a sink or bathtub while plugged in, it could cause a lethal shock. Unplug all small appliances when not in use.

YES ___ NO ___ 32. Are lamps or light switches within reach of each bed?

RECOMMENDATION: Lamps or switches located close to each bed will enable people getting up at night to see where they are going. Rearrange furniture closer to switches or move lamps closer to beds. Install night lights.

YES ___ NO ___ 33. Are ash trays, smoking materials, or other fire sources (heaters, hot plates, teapots, etc.) located away from beds or bedding?

RECOMMENDATION: Burns are a leading cause of accidental death among seniors. Smoking in bed is a major contributor to this problem. Remove sources of heat or flame from areas around beds. Don't smoke in bed.

YES ___ NO ___ 34. Is anything covering your electric blanket when in use?

RECOMMENDATION: "Tucking in" electric blankets, or placing additional coverings on top of them can cause excessive heat buildup which can start a fire.

YES ___ NO ___ 35. Do you ever go to sleep with a heating pad which is turned on?

RECOMMENDATION: Never go to sleep with a heating pad if it is turned on because it can cause serious burns even at relatively low settings.

YES ___ NO ___ 36. Is there a telephone close to your bed?

RECOMMENDATION: In case of an emergency, it is important to be able to reach the telephone without getting out of bed.

YES ___ NO ___ 37. Are work areas, especially areas where power tools are used, well lit?

RECOMMENDATION: Either install additional light, or avoid working with power tools in the area.

YES ___ NO ___ 38. Can you turn on the lights without first having to walk through a dark area?

RECOMMENDATION: Keep an operating flashlight handy. Have an electrician install switches at each entrance to a dark area.

YES ___ NO ___ 39. If fuses are used, are they the correct size for the circuit?

RECOMMENDATION: Replacing a correct size fuse with a larger size fuse can present a serious fire hazard.

YES ___ NO ___ 40. Are power tools equipped with a 3-prong plug or marked to show that they are double insulated?

RECOMMENDATION: These safety features reduce the risk of an electric shock. Use a properly connected 3-prong adapter for connecting a 3- prong plug to a 2-hole receptacle.

YES ___ NO ___ 41. Are power tools guards in place?

RECOMMENDATION: Power tools used with guards removed pose a serious risk of injury from sharp edges or moving parts.

YES ___ NO ___ 42. Are containers of volatile liquids tightly capped?

RECOMMENDATION: If not tightly closed, vapors may escape that may be toxic when inhaled. Check containers periodically to make sure they are tightly closed.

YES ___ NO ___ 43. Are gasoline, paints, solvents, or other products that give off vapors or fumes stored away from ignition sources?

RECOMMENDATION: Gasoline, kerosene, and other flammable liquids should be stored out of living areas in properly labeled, non- glass safety containers. Remove these products from the areas near heat or flame such as heaters, furnaces, water heaters, ranges, and other gas appliances.

YES ___ NO ___ 44. Are stairs well lighted?

RECOMMENDATION: Stairs should be lighted so that each step, particularly the step edges, can be clearly seen while going up and down stairs. The lighting should not produce glare or shadows along the stairway.

YES ____ NO ____ 45. Are light switches located at both the top and bottom of the stairs.

RECOMMENDATION: Install night lights at nearby outlets. Consider installing switches at the top and bottom of the stairs.

YES ___ NO ___ 46. Do the steps allow secure footing?

RECOMMENDATION: Worn treads or worn or loose carpeting can lead to insecure footing, resulting in slips or falls. Make certain the carpet is firmly attached to the steps all along the stairs.

YES ___ NO ___ 47. Are steps even and of the same size and height?

RECOMMENDATION: Even a small difference in step surfaces or riser heights can lead to falls. Mark any steps which are especially narrow or have risers that are higher or lower than the others. Be especially careful of these steps when using the stairs.

YES ___ NO ___ 48. Are the coverings on the steps in good condition?

RECOMMENDATION: Repair coverings. Remove coverings. Replace coverings.

YES ___ NO ___ 49. Can you clearly see the edges of the steps?

RECOMMENDATION: Falls may occur if the edges of the steps are blurred or hard to see. Paint edges of outdoor steps white to see them better at night. Add extra lighting.

YES ___ NO ___ 50. Is anything stored on the stairway, even temporarily?

RECOMMENDATION: Remove all objects from the stairway.

Source: U.S Consumer Product Safety Commission, Washington, D.C.

Characteristics of Perpetrators of Workplace Violence

Indicate whether or not you work with someone who exhibits the following characteristics.

Yes No Prior Verbal Threats: If the employee engages in threatening conduct toward other employees or supervisors, this threat should be taken seriously and the employer should respond in an appropriate manner.

Yes No Intimidating Behavior: The employee may exhibit any of the following behaviors: repeated phone calls to the victim, following the victim, and/or leaving messages for the victim.

Yes No Mental Health Problems: Depression, fantasies, irrational/violent thoughts, paranoid delusions, and extreme mood swings all may indicate a potential for workplace violence.

Yes No Obsessions: The employee may be preoccupied with weapons and/or the military, or hurting a specific person. He or she may believe a romantic attachment exists with a co-worker.

Yes No Decline in Performance: Recent excessive and unexplained absences from the job, concentration problems, increased signs of poor health or hygiene and the inability to accept responsibility for errors.

Yes No Stress: Increased stress in the employee's personal life including financial problems, problems in his or her marriage or other relationships, inappropriate display of emotions on the job such as uncontrolled anger or excessive crying.

Yes No Substance Abuse: Some drugs increase paranoia and others can cause aggressive behavior. Alcohol is present in many violent situations. While there is no scientific evidence to substantiate that substance abuse causes violence, it is present in many of the reported cases of violent behavior.

Scoring

For every "Yes" you circled, you have identified a common characteristic of those who commit violence in the workplace. These characteristics should give you reason to be more suspicious or careful in any given situation. However, law enforcement personnel still do not have the ability to predict violent behavior in certain specific situations. No definite profile has been accepted by the professionals in this area.

Source: <u>Workplace Violence: Its Nature and Extent</u>, Office for Victims of Crime, Office of Justice Programs, U.S. Department of Justice

Does She Have a Safety Plan?

On behalf of someone you know who is living in a battering environment, circle the response that indicates what preparations have been made to have a safety plan:

Yes	No	Does she have family and friends with whom she can stay?
Yes	No	Would she find a protective or restraining order helpful?
Yes	No	Can a victim advocate safely contact her at home? What should the advocate do if the batterer answers the phone?
Yes	No	Does she know how to contact emergency assistance (i.e. 911)?
Yes	No	If she believes the violence might begin or escalate, can she leave for a few days?
Yes	No	Does she know how to contact the shelter (if she doesn't, provide her with information for future use)?
Yes	No	Does she have a neighbor she can contact, or work out a signal for assistance, when violence erupts or appears inevitable?
Yes	No	If she has a car, can she hide a set of keys?
Yes	No	Can she pack an extra set of clothes for herself and the children, and store them – along with an extra set of house and car keys – with a neighbor or a friend?
Yes	No	Can she leave extra cash, checkbook or savings account book hidden or with a friend for emergency access?
Yes	No	Can she collect and store originals or copies of important records such as birth certificates, social security cards, her driver's license, financial records (such as banking and other financial accounts, mortgage or rent receipts, the title to the car, etc.), and medical records (for her children and herself)?
Yes	No	Does she have a concrete plan for exactly where she should go and how she can get there, at any time regardless of when she leaves?
Yes	No	Does she have a disability that requires assistance or a specialized safety plan?
Yes	No	Does she want access to counseling for her children or herself?

Scoring

Every "Yes" response indicates that progress is being made in terms of establishing a "safety plan." If and when a victim is able to leave her battering environment, it is essential that she has a "safety plan" to increase her opportunity for a successful departure. Advance planning is crucial.

Source: Developed from information provided in the 1998 National Victim Assistance Academy by J.N. Burnley, C. Edmunds, M.T. Gaboury, & A. Seymours (Eds.). Office for Victims of Crime, Office of Justice Programs, U.S. Department of Justice.

Can You Help Survivors of Homicide?

Indicate which of the following ways you would try to help a survivor of homicide:

Yes No 1. Allow survivors to grieve in whatever manner they wish and for as long as they wish.

Yes No 2. Allow survivors to cry freely. It is a healthy expression of grief and releases tensions.

Yes No 3. Allow survivors to talk about and personalize the victim. Let him or her tell you about the victim, his or her life and the murder. Allow the survivor to criticize the victim and to talk about the good times and the bad times.

Yes No 4. Say things like: "I understand." "It sounds like..." "I'm glad you can share those feelings." "You're lucky that...." "Don't worry, it's going to be alright."

Yes No 5. Allow survivors to get angry at you, the criminal justice system, the criminal, the victim, or simply the unfairness of life. Anger needs to be expressed.

Yes No 6. Remember the survivors at holiday times, on the anniversary date of the murder and the victim's birthday. Let the survivors know you remember, too.

Yes No 7. Allow the survivors some occasional "time out" from day-to-day pressures.

Yes No 8. Reassure the survivors that the murder was neither their fault, nor the victim's fault.

Yes No 9. Tell survivors that crime is simply a part of life and that they need to accept it.

Yes No 10. Support survivors in their efforts to reconstruct a life, even if it means a major change in lifestyle.

Yes No 11. Let survivors know that you will remain their friend and they mean a great deal to you.

Yes No 12. Make sure the victims/survivors feel safe and/or secure.

Yes No 13. Give victims permission to express any reactions and respond in a non-judgmental manner. Say: "You have a right to be upset over this tragedy, so don't be afraid to tell me what you are thinking."

Yes No 14. Respond to the victim's need for nurturing by allowing the victim to become dependent.

Yes No 15. Initially take care of practical things that need to be done, but are temporarily beyond the victim's ability to accomplish.

Yes No 16. Offer to provide child care, help with transportation, make telephone calls, etc. Be specific in making such offers so that the victim can simply respond "yes" or "no."

Yes No 17. Assist survivors in re-establishing a sense of control over the small things in his or her life, then move on to larger ones.

Yes No 18. Ask the victim to describe his or her reaction and responses. As the victim begins the description, validate the reactions and responses.

Yes No 19. Ask the victim to describe what has happened since the crime, including contact with family members, friends, the criminal justice system, and so on.

Yes No 20. Ask the victim to describe other reactions he or she has experienced up to now. Then, validate reactions.

Yes No 21. Let the victim talk for as long as he or she would like and as your time allows for you to listen.

Yes No 22. Say things like: "You are safe now" (if true). "I am sorry it happened." "I'm glad you're talking with me now."

Yes No 23. Don't assume anything, even if the apparent pattern of the crisis reaction is suspect. (For example, the victim's controlled calm of the moment may yield to tears in a few minutes.)

Scoring

"Yes" responses to items 1 - 3, 5 - 8, and 10 - 13, 15 - 23 and "No" responses to items 4, 9 and 14, indicate that you can be helpful to survivors of homicide.

Source: Developed from information provided in the 1998 National Victim Assistance Academy by Jane N. Burnley, Christine Edmunds, Mario T. Gaboury, and Anne Seymour (Eds.). Office for Victims of Crime, Office of Justice Programs, U.S. Department of Justice

Types of Love

Name: ______________________________ Date: ____________

Directions: Read these descriptions carefully. How have you either given or received each of these types of love? Write down the occasions when you have been the source or recipient of each type of love, or write down the first names of people you have been involved with for each type of love. Can these types of love be combined?

Type of Love	Given To	Received From
Romantic Love	____________	____________
	____________	____________
	____________	____________
Possessive Love	____________	____________
	____________	____________
	____________	____________
Best Friends Love	____________	____________
	____________	____________
	____________	____________
Pragmatic Love	____________	____________
	____________	____________
	____________	____________
Altruistic Love	____________	____________
	____________	____________
	____________	____________
Game-Playing Love	____________	____________
	____________	____________
	____________	____________

Are You and Your Partner Suited for a Life Together?

Name: ______________________________ Date: __________

Purpose: Most people carry an image in their hearts of the "perfect" marriage--marriage as they would wish it to be. But it can be hard to articulate. It is not always possible to state explicitly what it is you want...dream...wish...especially if you are not really sure yourself. And sometimes, it spoils everything when you have to ask for it.

Directions: Below you will find an inventory divided into ten areas. In the blanks provided to the right of each statement, you and your partner should answer either AGREE or DISAGREE or NEUTRAL to each statement.

COMMUNICATION	You	Partner
1. Let's share our experiences; ask me what I've been doing and tell me what you've been doing.	________	________
2. I'd like to be able to express my feelings without fear of criticism.	________	________
3. You shouldn't talk so much.	________	________
4. You shouldn't assume what I need without finding out first if you're right.	________	________
5. You shouldn't moralize.	________	________
6. Never lie to me.	________	________
7. I'd like you to guess what I need without having to tell you.	________	________
8. I wish you would learn to listen to me.	________	________
9. You can yell sometimes.	________	________
10. I don't like you to interrupt me.	________	________

DECISIONS		
1. I'd like to be the one who makes the important decisions.	________	________
2. Let's talk over everything and always make joint decisions.	________	________
3. I am ready to lie, bribe, and blackmail just to get my way.	________	________
4. Let's agree in advance who's to make decisions in each area of our lives together.	________	________
5. Let's try to persuade each other quietly and rationally.	________	________
6. When we disagree on major issues let's turn to somebody more experienced for help.	________	________

7. We should try to give in without trying to "get back" at each other. ______ ______
8. When we disagree, we should flip a coin in order to reach a decision. ______ ______
9. I want you to have the responsibility for making our decisions. ______ ______
10. In order to stay together, we should agree on everything. ______ ______

RELATIVES

1. I'd like to spend more time with my family. ______ ______
2. I would like our parents to help us out financially. ______ ______
3. I don't like you to criticize my family. ______ ______
4. I'd like to live near my parents. ______ ______
5. You should be nicer to my parents. ______ ______
6. We should spend our holidays with my family. ______ ______
7. You consult your parents too frequently. ______ ______
8. Don't compare me to your mother/father. ______ ______
9. I'd like your parents not to interfere in our lives. ______ ______
10. We should consult our parents on important issues. ______ ______

ROLES

1. We should divide chores equally between us. ______ ______
2. My career should come first. ______ ______
3. You should plan our social life. ______ ______
4. You should be the one to invite friends over. ______ ______
5. You should be responsible for the children's education. ______ ______
6. I'll be responsible for the yard and garden work. ______ ______
7. You should be responsible for household repairs. ______ ______
8. My job is to earn a living for the family. ______ ______
9. I'll be responsible for decorating our home. ______ ______
10. We'll share the cooking between us. ______ ______

CONFLICTS

1. We should never quarrel. ______ ______
2. You should be the first to make up. ______ ______
3. You should learn to control your emotions. ______ ______
4. I don't like you to run away in the middle of a fight. ______ ______
5. We should always make up before we go to bed. ______ ______
6. During a quarrel, we should be allowed to curse. ______ ______
7. When we argue, we shouldn't bring up grievances from the past. ______ ______
8. It's all right to cry during a quarrel. ______ ______
9. It's all right to yell and let off steam when we argue. ______ ______
10. We should always keep our anger under control. ______ ______

ENTERTAINMENT

1. We should spend all our free time together. ______ ______
2. We must invite friends over at least once a week. ______ ______
3. We should get out of the house quite often and go to a movie, play, concert, or just out to dinner. ______ ______
4. Once a year we should go on a special vacation together. ______ ______
5. I'd like to have time on my own at least once a week. ______ ______
6. We should take time every day to talk things over and be together. ______ ______
7. You shouldn't spend so much time sleeping when we are together. ______ ______
8. I need to have enough time alone to spend on my hobbies. ______ ______
9. We should have a large circle of friends. ______ ______
10. I want to spend as much time as possible at home. ______ ______

AFFECTION

1. You should often tell me you love me. ______ ______
2. I would like you to hug and caress me a lot. ______ ______
3. It's OK for us to show affection in public. ______ ______

4. I'd like you to give me a gift from time to time, not just on birthdays or anniversaries. ______ ______
5. You should tell me more often that I'm attractive. ______ ______
6. You should always remember my birthday/our anniversary. ______ ______
7. From time to time, I'd like to act out romantic fantasies together. ______ ______
8. I like it when you dance only with me at parties. ______ ______
9. I like you to baby me from time to time. ______ ______
10. I'd like you to take me in your arms and comfort me when I'm sad. ______ ______

MONEY

1. We should have separate bank accounts. ______ ______
2. We should plan all our household expenses together. ______ ______
3. You should be responsible for paying monthly bills. ______ ______
4. I'll decide what our expenses should be. ______ ______
5. I don't want to have to report to you every time I spend money. ______ ______
6. We should each have some money for our personal use, to spend any way we choose. ______ ______
7. We should put every spare penny into a savings account. ______ ______
8. We should keep a monthly record of expenses. ______ ______
9. We should make only cash purchases and not buy credit. ______ ______
10. We should spend our money as we please, enjoying today and not worrying about tomorrow. ______ ______

SEX

1. You should initiate sex. ______ ______
2. You should be able to guess what makes me feel good. ______ ______
3. We should have sex more often. ______ ______
4. We should have sex only when I show signs that I really want it. ______ ______
5. Our sex life should be varied. ______ ______

6. You should not feel rejected or try to make me feel guilty when I'm not in the mood to make love. __________ __________
7. You should never desire anyone else. __________ __________
8. You should feel free to have an affair. __________ __________
9. You should tell me if you have an affair. __________ __________
10. You should be responsible for birth control. __________ __________

PARENTHOOD

Note: If you do not have--or plan to have--children answer "as if" you do, to questions 5-10.

1. We should have only "planned" children. __________ __________
2. We should postpone having children until we have established our careers and are prepared financially. __________ __________
3. It's a mother's duty to stay home to bring up the children. __________ __________
4. We will have no children. __________ __________
5. We should always keep a united front and never argue in front of our children. __________ __________
6. Our children's needs should always come before our own. __________ __________
7. Our children should be punished when they are bad. __________ __________
8. Our children should grow up free from any restrictions. __________ __________
9. Our children should have everything we could not have as children. __________ __________
10. Whatever happens, we should stay together for the children's sake until they are grown. __________ __________

Scoring: Now compare your answers. For each "compatible" answer, score 1 point. There are several ways to arrive at a compatible score, so a discussion period aimed at determining compatibility is very important.

For example: You have a compatible answer if you both gave the same answer to a statement such as "Let's talk over everything and always make joint decisions."

However, you also have a compatible answer if one of you answers "Disagree" to such a statement as "I'd like to be the one to make the important decisions" (this person does not want to make the decisions). Therefore, if the other partner answered "Agree" to the same statement, the one person's objection is compatible with the other's agreement with the statement.

A third example is where both of you have answered "Neutral" to an item; your choice is compatible since the issue is not important to either of you. Even if one of you answered "Neutral" and the other answered either "Agree" or "Disagree," communication about the issue involved may determine whether your attitudes are in conflict. One of you may even change your original choice, if the issue--after discussion--fades (or increases) in importance. Being able to arrive at an answer through this discussion indicates compatibility.

After discussing your answers with your partner, total your "compatibility" answers for each questionnaire. List them here:

Communication	____
Decisions	____
Relatives	____
Roles	____
Conflicts	____
Entertainment	____
Affection	____
Money	____
Sex	____
Parenthood	____
TOTAL	____

Analysis:

Score	Compatibility Prognosis
Below 10	You had better part on friendly terms right now (if you haven't already done so while answering the questionnaires). You are not suited for a life together.
11 to 50	Each one of you is a distinct individual, with different ambitions and goals. However, this does not mean that you cannot live happily together if you do not mistake interference for intimacy. Keep your distinct worlds.
51 to 90	You are well matched but should re-examine the issues you disagree on. Try to reach a common denominator.
91 and up	You suit each other perfectly and stand a good chance for a long and happy life together.

Source: Robert F. Valois and Sandra Kammerman. Your Sexuality: A Self- Assessment, 2nd Ed. New York McGraw-Hill, 1992: 212-217.

Getting to Know Your Own Level of Trust

Name: ______________________ Date: __________

Directions: Reach each of the following statements and decide whether it is true of your relationship with your partner. Indicate how strongly you agree or disagree by choosing the appropriate number from the scale below and placing it in the space provided in the left-hand margin.

1 = strongly disagree	5 = mildly agree
2 = moderately disagree	6 = moderately agree
3 = mildly disagree	7 = strongly agree
4 = neutral	

Initial Score *Final Score*

___ 1. I know how my partner is going to act. May partner can always be counted on to act as I expect. ___

___ 2. I have found that my partner is a thoroughly dependable person, especially when it comes to things that are important. ___

___ 3. My partner's behavior tends to be quite variable. I can't always be sure what my partner will surprise me with next. ___

___ 4. Though times may change and the future in uncertain, I have faith that my partner will always be ready and willing to offer me strength, come what may. ___

___ 5. Based on past experience, I cannot with complete confidence, rely on my partner to keep promises made to me. ___

___ 6. It is sometimes difficult for me to be absolutely certain that my partner will always continue to care for me; the future holds too many uncertainties and too many things can change in our relationship as time goes on. ___

___ 7. My partner is a very honest person and, even if my partner were to make unbelievable statements, people should feel confident that what they are hearing is the truth. ___

___ 8. My partner is not very predictable. People can't always be certain how my partner is going to act from one day to another. ___

___ 9. My partner has proven to be a faithful person. No matter who my partner was married to, she or he would never be unfaithful, even if there was absolutely no chance of being caught. ___

___ 10. I am never concerned that unpredictable conflicts and serious tensions may damage our relationship because I know we can weather any storm. ___

___ 11. I am very familiar with the patterns of behavior my partner has established, and he or she will behave in certain ways. ___

___ 12. If I have never faced a particular issue with my partner before, I occasionally worry that he or she won't take my feelings into account. ___

___ 13. Even in familiar circumstances, I am not totally certain my partner will act in the same way twice. ___

Initial Score		*Final Score*
___	14. I feel completely secure in facing unknown new situations because I know my partner will never let me down.	___
___	15. My partner is not necessarily someone others always consider reliable. I can think of some times when my partner could not be counted on.	___
___	16. I occasionally find myself feeling uncomfortable with the emotional investment I have made in our relationship because I find it hard to completely set aside my doubts about what lies ahead.	___
___	17. My partner has not always proven to be trustworthy in the past, and there are times when I am hesitant to let my partner engage in activities that make me feel vulnerable.	___
___	18. My partner behaves in a consistent manner.	___

Scoring: This is how to score yourself: For questions 3, 5, 6, 8, 12, 13, 15, 16 and 17, reverse numbers. That is, if you put down a 1, change it to a 7, and write this in the space provided in the right-hand margin. In the same way, if you scored a 2 change it to a 6, 3 to a 5, 5 to a 3, 6 to a 2, and 7 to a 1. A neutral score of 4 remains unchanged.

When you have reversed the scoring for the items listed above, take the scores for the remaining items and write them in the right-hand margin just as they are. Add all the scores in the right-hand margin to obtain your final trust score.

If you are interested, you can add up the scores for the following questions to arrive at a score for each subscale of trust: Predictability, add 1, 3, 8, 11, 13, and 18. Dependability, add 2, 5, 7, 9, 15, and 17. Faith, add 4, 6, 10, 12, 14, and 16.

Source: John Rempel and John Holmes, 1986 "How Do I Trust Thee?" Psychology Today (February): 30-31. Reprinted with permission from Psychology Today Magazine.

Needs In Close Relationships

Name: ______________________________ Date: ____________

Check one: I want my boy friend to ... I want my girl friend to ...
I want my husband to ... I want my wife to ...

Directions: Choose from the list below the affectional needs you feel the strongest.

___ 1. Allow me more freedom.
___ 2. Display more affection for me.
___ 3. Have more respect for my judgment.
___ 4. Feel more attached to me.
___ 5. Treat me in a warmer and friendlier manner.
___ 6. Be more interested in my activities.
___ 7. Take me out more.
___ 8. Engage more in activities with me.
___ 9. Allow me to make more decisions.
___ 10. Display more love for me.
___ 11. Feel more strongly that I am a significant aspect of his/her life.
___ 12. Have more respect for my ability to think for myself.
___ 13. Share more of his/her recreational time with me.
___ 14. Expect less accomplishment from me.
___ 15. Be more interested in me.
___ 16. Be warmer and closer in his/her behavior toward me.
___ 17. Feel more strongly that I am an important member of the family.
___ 18. Have more confidence in my ability to learn things.
___ 19. Spend more time with me.
___ 20. Give me more freedom to choose my own friends.
___ 21. Be more interested in the things I'm interested in.
___ 22. Spend more time alone with me.
___ 23. Put fewer limits on what I do.
___ 24. Give me more praise for my accomplishments.
___ 25. Be more confident that I will succeed in life.
___ 26. Give me more attention.
___ 27. Feel more love for me.
___ 28. Be more interested in being with me around the house.
___ 29. Feel more confident about my ability to think critically.

___ 30. Allow me to think for myself.

___ 31. Feel closer to me as a person.

___ 32. Feel more strongly that I am significant person.

___ 33. Have more respect for my ability to solve problems.

___ 34. Take me out more/go on more trips with me.

___ 35. Criticize me less for my conduct and manners.

___ 36. Feel more strongly that I am an important person.

___ 37. Feel more confident about my ability to succeed at difficult tasks.

___ 38. Spend more of his/her free time with me.

___ 39. Supervise my activities less.

___ 40. Feel more affection for me.

___ 41. Be more confident that I can be trusted with responsibilities.

___ 42. Spend more time showing me how to do certain things.

___ 43. Insist less on respect from me.

___ 44. Feel more warmth for me.

___ 45. Display more romantic love and/or sexual passion with me.

Describe your needs in a close relationship.

Muehlenhard-Quackenbush Sexual Attitude Scale

Name: ______________________________ Date: __________

Purpose: This exercise is designed for you and your partner or friend to examine some of their attitudes about male and female sexuality.

Directions: Reach each of the statements below carefully and respond using the scale provided.

A = Agree Strongly   B = Agree Mildly   C = Disagree Mildly   D = Disagree Strongly

	You	Partner/ Friend
1. It's worse for a woman to sleep around than it is for a man.	____	____
2. It's best for a guy to lose his virginity before he's out of his teens.	____	____
3. It's okay for a woman to have more than one sexual relationship at a time.	____	____
4. It is just as important for a man to be a virgin when he marries as it is for a woman.	____	____
5. I approve of a 16-year-old girl having sex just as much as a 16-year-old boy having sex.	____	____
6. I kind of admire a girl who has had sex with a lot of guys.	____	____
7. I kind of feel sorry for a 21-year-old woman who is still a virgin.	____	____
8. A woman having casual sex is just as acceptable to me as a man having casual sex.	____	____
9. It's ok for a man to have sex with a woman he is not in love with.	____	____
10. I kind of admire a guy who has had sex with a lot of girls.	____	____
11. A woman who initiates sex is too aggressive.	____	____
12. It's ok for a man to have more than one sexual relationship at a time.	____	____
13. I question the character of a woman who has had a lot of sexual partners.	____	____
14. I admire a man who is a virgin when he gets married.	____	____
15. A man should be more sexually experienced than his wife.	____	____
16. A girl who has sex on the first date is easy.	____	____
17. I kind of feel sorry for a 21-year-old man who is still a virgin.	____	____

	You	Partner/ Friend
18. I question the character of a guy who has had a lot of sexual partners.	____	____
19. Women are naturally more monogamous (inclined to stick to one partner) than are men.	____	____
20. A man should be sexually experienced when he gets married.	____	____
21. A guy who has sex on the first date is easy.	____	____
22. It's ok for a woman to have sex with a man she is not in love with.	____	____
23. A woman should be sexually experienced when she gets married.	____	____
24. It's best for a girl to lose her virginity before she's out of her teens.	____	____
25. I admire a women who is a virgin when she gets married.	____	____
26. A man who initiates sex is too aggressive.	____	____

Scoring: Convert your A's to zeros, your B's to 1's, your C's to 2's, your D's to 3's. Computing your total involves some simple mathematics:

#4 + #5 + #8 + (3 - #1) + (3 - #15) + (3 - #19) + (#24 - #2) + (#3 - #12) + (#6 - #10) + (#7 - #17) + (#22 - #9) + (#26 - #11) + (#18 - #13) + (#14 - #25) + (21 - #16) + (#23 - #20) = YOUR TOTAL

Interpretation: The actual name of the scale is the Sexual Double Standard Scale. A person having identical sexual standards for women and men should score zero. A score greater than zero reflects more restrictive sexual standards for women than for men; the highest possible score is 48. A score less than zero reflects more restrictive sexual standards for men than for women; the lowest possible score is -30.

From a sample of college students at a large southwestern university, researchers found a mean score for women to be 11.99 (N=461) and a mean score for men to be 13.15 (N=255).

Source: Charlene L. Muehlenhard and Debra M. Quackenbush The Sexual Double Standard Scale, Department of Psychology and Women's Studies University of Kansas. Reprinted with permission.

Index of Sexual Satisfaction

Name: ______________________________________ Date: ___________

Directions: For each of the following statements, assign a number reflecting your current or past sexual relationships as follows:

1 = Rarely or none of the time
2 = A little of the time
3 = Some of the time
4 = A good part of the time
5 = Most or all of the time

___ 1. I feel that my partner enjoys our sex life.

___ 2. My sex life is very exciting.

___ 3. Sex is fun for my partner and me.

___ 4. I feel that my partner sees little in me except for the sex I can give.

___ 5. I feel that sex is dirty and disgusting.

___ 6. My sex life is monotonous.

___ 7. When we have sex it is too rushed and hurriedly completed.

___ 8. I feel that my sex life is lacking quality.

___ 9. My partner is very sexually exciting.

___ 10. I enjoy the sex techniques that my partner likes or uses.

___ 11. I feel that my partner wants too much sex from me.

___ 12. I think that sex is wonderful.

___ 13. My partner dwells on sex too much.

___ 14. I feel that sex is something that has to be endured in our relationship.

___ 15. My partner is too rough or brutal when we have sex.

___ 16. My partner observes good personal hygiene.

___ 17. I feel that sex is a normal function of our relationship.

___ 18. My partner does not want sex when I do.

___ 19. I feel that our sex life really adds a lot to our relationship.

___ 20. I would like to have sexual contact with someone other than my partner.

___ 21. It is easy for me to get sexually excited by my partner.

___ 22. I feel that my partner is sexually pleased with me.

___ 23. My partner is very sensitive to my sexual needs and desires.

___ 24. I feel that I should have sex more often.

___ 25. I feel that my sex life is boring.

Scoring: Use the following key to score your answers:

- Score number answered for questions 4, 5, 6, 7, 8, 11, 13, 14, 15, 18, 20, 24, and 25.
- Score reverse of number answered (see below) for questions 1, 2, 3, 9, 10, 12, 16, 17, 19, 21, 22, and 23.
- To score the reverse of number answered:
  if you answered "1," score 5
  if you answered "2," score 4
  if you answered "3," score 3
  if you answered "4," score 2
  if you answered "5," score 1

Interpretation:

0–29 You have little dissatisfaction with your sex life and enjoy a mutually enjoyable and stimulating sex life, probably in a long-lasting relationship.

30-100 You are somewhat to very dissatisfied with your sex life and may be involved in a disintegrating relationship.

Source: Rita Aero and Elliot Weiner The Mind Test New York: William Morrow & Co., 1981.

Love and Sex

Name: ______________________________ Date: __________

Directions: Complete the following sentence by writing down your immediate thoughts. Do not think too much about your response.

1. Love is ______________________________.
2. My greatest fear of love is ______________________________.
3. To me, love without sex is ______________________________.
4. To me, love with sex is ______________________________.
5. To me, sex without love is ______________________________.
6. I need love because ______________________________.
7. I feel most loved when ______________________________.
8. One lovable quality about me is ______________________________ ______________________________.
9. I could increase my ability to love others by ______________________________.
10. I express my love for others primarily by ______________________________.
11. To me love means ______________________________.
12. If nobody loved me, ______________________________.
13. For me the greatest risk in loving is ______________________________.
14. When I'm with those I love, I ______________________________ ______________________________.
15. When I'm separated from my loved ones, I ______________________________ ______________________________.

Parents? Inventory

Name: ______________________________ Date: ____________

Purpose: Because two people are needed to conceive a child, two people should determine whether and when to conceive. The advent of more reliable birth control makes such planning possible. If you are considering having a child, this exercise will help you examine the expectations that you and your partner have of parenthood. Even if you feel parenthood is far off in the future, this will help you determine your current expectations.

Directions: You and your partner should independently write a sentence or two in answer to each question. Then go through what you have written and indicate, by a check in the proper column, whether each of these predictions would make you pleased, unhappy, or neither if it came true. Pick out which of the areas covered in the questions are most important to you in your decision. (If you do not have a partner, ask a friend to complete the inventory. This will give you a perspective of differences of opinion that can be involved and the complexity of the issue.)

Assessment

	Pleased	Unhappy	Neither
1. How will having a child affect my partner's and/or my career and/or education?	_____	_____	_____
2. How will a child affect our financial situation now and later?	_____	_____	_____
3. How will the child affect our relationship with each other?	_____	_____	_____
4. How will the child affect our relationship with family and friends?	_____	_____	_____
5. How will the child affect our freedom, privacy, and spontaneity?	_____	_____	_____
6. How will my partner and I deal with the pregnancy and birth?	_____	_____	_____
7. How will each of us deal with supervising, training, and being with a young child (birth to 8 years)?	_____	_____	_____
8. How will we deal with supervising, training and being with an older child or teenager?	_____	_____	_____
9. How will we deal with possible problems of health and personality our child could have?	_____	_____	_____
10. How do we feel about bringing up a child in today's world (i.e., what kinds of problems and solutions are there for the child's future world)?	_____	_____	_____

Scoring: Compare answers with your partner. Discussing realistic predictions of parenthood can quell some fears (or bring others to mind) and be a starting point for making a decision.

Personal Application: The following worksheet will help you think through the impact a child will have on your life. In the first column list needs you have that a child might help satisfy--for example, the need for love, for attention, and for alleviation of boredom. Then, in the second column, list other ways these same needs could be met.

NEEDS A CHILD COULD SATISFY	OTHER WAYS THESE NEEDS COULD BE MET
____________________	____________________
____________________	____________________
____________________	____________________
____________________	____________________

NEEDS A CHILD COULD SATISFY	OTHER WAYS THESE NEEDS COULD BE MET
____________________	____________________
____________________	____________________
____________________	____________________
____________________	____________________

List reasons for choosing to have a child. These can range from very personal reasons to reasons having to do with external factors.

1. ____________________
2. ____________________
3. ____________________
4. ____________________
5. ____________________
6. ____________________
7. ____________________

List disadvantages of having children.

1. ____________________
2. ____________________
3. ____________________
4. ____________________

Source: Blake et al, Self-Assessment and Behavior Change Manual. New York: Random House, 1984. 84-86.

Should You Have the HIV Test?

Directions
Indicate whether or not you have engaged in any of the following behaviors:

Yes No 1. I have had sex without knowing for sure if the person or persons you had sex with do not have HIV?

Yes No 2. I have had sex with someone you know has HIV or AIDS?

Yes No 3. I have had a disease passed on by sex, like genital herpes or syphilis? (Having these diseases makes it easier to get HIV.)

Yes No 4. I have had sex with many men or women or had sex with someone who has

Yes No 5. I have had sex with many men or women?

Yes No 6. I have had sex with someone who has used needles to take drugs?

Yes No 7. I have shared needles or works to take drugs?

Scoring
If you have answered "yes" to any of these questions, you should think about being tested for HIV.

Source: Adapted from "Should You Have the HIV Test?" How to Help Yourself Series, National Institute of Allergy and Infectious Diseases, National Institutes of Health

Are You Ready for a Healthy Pregnancy?

Indicate which behaviors match your own or your female partner's behaviors:

	Done	Will Do	Won't Do
1. Get a physical exam			
2. Reduce your use of tobacco, alcohol, caffeine, and non-prescription drugs.			
3. Get to an optimal weight.			
4. Establish a well balanced, nutritious diet that includes plenty of folic acid.			
5. Maintain a regular exercise routine.			
6. Talk to your health care professional about any chronic medical conditions you might have.			
7. Get any necessary vaccinations.			
8. If you are using a hormonal contraceptive method, change to another method.			
9. If you are a cat owner, make arrangements for someone else to deal with the kitty litter.			
10. Avoid any exposure to X-rays.			
11. Avoid extremes in body temperature (e.g., hot tubs).			
TOTAL			

Scoring

A total of 11 for the "Done" column indicates that you (or your female partner) are in a good position healthwise to begin attempting to become pregnant. (Remember, however, that this survey does not replace the need for seeing a physician to truly determine your readiness.) Points in the "Will Do" column total indicate that you are contemplating steps to take to ensure a healthy pregnancy. Any points in the "Won't Do" column total indicate that you are failing to take precautions necessary for a healthy pregnancy.

Source: "From Data to Action," CDC's Public Health Surveillance for Women, Infants and Children

Rating Your Diet

Name: ______________________________ Date: ____________

Purpose: The 40 questions which follow will help you focus on the key features of your diet. The (+) or (-) numbers under each set of answers instantly pat you on the back for good habits or alert you to problems you may not have realized you have.

The Grand Total rates your overall diet, on a scale from "Great" to "Arghh!"

The quiz focuses on fat, cholesterol, sodium, sugar, fiber, and vitamins A and C. It doesn't attempt to cover everything in your diet. Also, it doesn't try to measure precisely how much of these key nutrients you eat.

What the quiz will do is give you a rough sketch of your current eating habits and, implicitly, suggest what you can do to improve them.

Finally, please don't despair over a less-than-perfect score. A healthy diet isn't built overnight.

Directions:

- o Next to each answer is a number with a + or - sign in front of it. Circle the number that is directly next to the answer you choose. That's your score for the question. (If you use a pencil, you can erase your answers and give the quiz to someone else.)
- o Circle only one number for each question, unless the instructions tell you to "average two or more scores if necessary."
- o How to average: In answering question 18, for example, if you drink club soda (+3) and coffee (-1) on a typical day, add the two scores (which gives you +2) and then divide by 2. That gives you a score of +1 for the question. If averaging gives you a fraction, round it to the nearest whole number.
- o If a question doesn't apply to you, skip it.
- o Pay attention to serving sizes. For example, a serving of vegetables is 1/2 cup. If you usually eat one cup of vegetables at a time, count it as two servings.
- o Add up all your + scores and your - scores.
- o Subtract your - scores from your + scores. That's your GRAND TOTAL.

1. How many times per week do you eat unprocessed red meat (steak, roast beef, lamb, or pork chops, burgers, etc.)?

(a) never	+3	(d) 4-5	-1
(b) 1 or less	+2	(e) 6 or more	-3
(c) 2-3	0		

2. After cooking, how large is the serving of red meat you usually eat? *(To convert from raw to cooked, reduce by 25 percent. For example, 4 oz. of raw meat shrinks to 3 oz. after cooking. There are 16 oz. in a pound.)*

(a) 8 oz. or more	-3	(d) 3 oz. or less	0
(b) 6-7 oz.	-2	(e) don't eat red meat	+3
(c) 4-5 oz.	-1		

3. Do you trim the visible fat when you cook or eat red meat?
(a) yes +1
(b) no -3
(c) don't eat red meat 0

4. How many times per week do you eat processed meats (hot dogs, bacon, sausage, bologna, luncheon meats, etc.)? *(OMIT products that contain one gram of fat or less per serving.)*
(a) none +3
(b) less than 1 +2
(c) 1-2 0
(d) 3-4 -1
(e) 5 or more -3

5. What kind of ground meat or poultry do you usually eat?
(a) regular ground beef -3
(b) lean ground beef -2
(c) ground round 0
(d) ground turkey +1
(e) Healthy Choice +2
(f) don't eat ground meat +3

6. What type of bread do you usually eat?
(a) whole wheat or other whole grain +3
(b) rye +2
(c) pumpernickel +2
(d) white, "wheat" French or Italian -1

7. How many times per week do you eat deep-fried foods (fish, chicken, vegetables, potatoes, etc.)?
(a) none +3
(b) 1-2 0
(c) 3-4 -1
(d) 5 or more -3

8. How many servings of nonfried vegetables do you usually eat per day? *(One serving = 1/2 cup. INCLUDE potatoes.)*
(a) none -3
(b) 1 0
(c) 2 +1
(d) 3 +2
(e) 4 or more +3

9. How many servings of cruciferous vegetables do you usually eat per week? *(ONLY count kale, broccoli, cauliflower, cabbage, Brussels sprouts, greens, bok choy, kohlrabi, turnip, and rutabaga. One serving = 1/2 cup.)*
(a) none -3
(b) 1-3 +1
(c) 4-6 +2
(d) 7 or more +3

10. How many servings of vitamin-A-rich fruits or vegetables do you usually eat per week? *(ONLY count carrots, pumpkin, sweet potatoes, cantaloupe, spinach, winter squash, greens, and apricots. One serving = 1/2 cup.)*
(a) none -3
(b) 1-3 +1
(c) 4-6 +2
(d) 7 or more +3

11. How many times per week do you eat at a fastfood restaurant? *(INCLUDE burgers, fried fish or chicken, croissant or biscuit sandwiches, topped potatoes, and other main dishes. OMIT meals of just plain baked potato, broiled chicken, or salad.)*
(a) never +3
(b) less than 1 +1
(c) 1 0
(d) 2 -1
(e) 3 -2
(f) 4 or more -3

12. How many servings of grains rich in complex carbohydrates do you eat per day? *(One serving = 1 slice of bread, 1 large pancake, 1 cup whole grain cold cereal, or 1/2 cup cooked cereal, rice, pasta, bulgur, wheat berries, kasha, or millet. OMIT heavily-sweetened cold cereals.)*
(a) none -3
(b) 1-3 0
(c) 4-5 +1
(d) 6-8 +2
(e) 9 or more +3

13. How many times per week do you eat fish or shellfish? *(OMIT deep-fried items, tuna packed in oil, shrimp, squid, and mayonnaise--laden tuna salad--a little mayo is okay.)*
(a) never -2
(b) 1-2 +1
(c) 3-4 +2
(d) 5 or more +3

14. How many times per week do you eat cheese? *(INCLUDE pizza, cheeseburgers, veal or eggplant parmigiana, cream cheese, etc. OMIT low-fat or fat-free cheeses.)*
(a) 1 or less +3
(b) 2-3 +2
(c) 4-5 -1
(d) 6 or more -3

15. How many servings of fresh fruit do you eat per day?
(a) none -3
(b) 1 0
(c) 2 +1
(d) 3 +2
(e) 4 or more +3

16. Do you remove the skin before eating poultry?
(a) Yes +3
(b) No -3
(c) don't eat poultry 0

17. What do you usually put on your bread or toast? *(AVERAGE two or more scores if necessary.)*
(a) butter or cream cheese -3
(b) margarine or peanut butter -2
(c) diet margarine -1
(d) jam or honey 0
(e) fruit butter +1
(f) nothing +3

18. Which of these beverages do you drink on a typical day? *(AVERAGE two or more scores if necessary.)*
(a) water or club soda +3
(b) fruit juice +1
(c) diet soda -1
(d) coffee or tea -3
(e) soda, fruit "drink", or fruit "ade" -3

19. Which flavorings do you most frequently add to your foods? *(AVERAGE two or more scores if necessary.)*
(a) garlic or lemon juice +3
(b) herbs or spices +3
(c) salt or soy sauce -2
(d) margarine -2
(e) butter -3
(f) nothing +3

20. What do you eat most frequently as a snack? *(AVERAGE two or more scores if necessary.)*
(a) fruits or vegetables +3
(b) sweetened yogurt +2
(c) nuts -1
(d) cookies or fried chips -2
(e) granola bar -2
(f) candy bar or pastry -3
(g) nothing 0

21. What is your most typical breakfast? *(SUBTRACT an extra 3 points if you also eat bacon or sausage.)*
(a) croissant, danish, or doughnut -3
(b) eggs -3
(c) pancakes or waffles -2
(d) cereal or toast +3
(e) low-fat yogurt or cottage cheese +3
(f) don't eat breakfast 0

22. What do you usually eat for dessert?
(a) pie, pastry, or cake -3
(b) ice cream -3
(c) fat-free cookies or cakes -1
(d) frozen yogurt or ice milk +1
(e) nonfat ice cream or sorbet +1
(f) fruit +3
(g) don't eat dessert +3

23. How many times per week do you eat beans, split peas, or lentils?
(a) none -2
(b) 1 +1
(c) 2 +2
(d) 3 or more +3

24. What kind of milk do you drink?
(a) whole -3
(b) 2% low-fat -1
(c) 1% low-fat +2
(d) 1/2% or skim +3
(e) none 0

25. What dressings or toppings do you usually add to your salads? *(ADD two or more scores if necessary.)*
(a) nothing, lemon or vinegar +3
(b) fat-free dressing +2
(c) low-or reduced-calorie dressing +1
(d) regular dressing -1
(e) croutons or bacon bits -1
(f) cole slaw, pasta salad, or potato salad -1

26. What sandwich filling do you eat most frequently? *(AVERAGE two or more scores if necessary.)*
(a) luncheon meat -3
(b) cheese or roast beef -1
(c) peanut butter 0
(d) low-fat luncheon meat +1
(e) tuna, salmon, chicken, or turkey +3
(f) don't eat sandwiches 0

27. What do you usually spread on your sandwiches? *(AVERAGE two or more scores if necessary.)*
(a) mayonnaise -2
(b) light mayonnaise -1
(c) catsup, mustard, or fat-free mayonnaise -0
(d) nothing +2

28. How many egg yolks do you eat per week? *(ADD 1 yolk for every slice of quiche you eat.)*
(a) 2 or less +3
(b) 3-4 0
(c) 5-6 -1
(d) 7 or more -3

29. How many times per week do you eat canned or dried soups? *(OMIT low-sodium, low-fat soups.)*

(a) none +3 (c) 3-4 -2
(b) 1-2 0 (d) 5 or more -3

30. How many servings of a rich source of calcium do you eat per day? *(One serving = 2/3 cup milk or yogurt, 1 oz. cheese, 1 1/2 oz. sardines, 3 1/2 oz. salmon, 5 oz. tofu made with calcium sulfate, 1 cup greens or broccoli, or 200 mg of a calcium supplement.)*

(a) none -3 (c) 2 +2
(b) 1 +1 (d) 3 or more +3

31. What do you usually order on your pizza? *(Vegetable toppings include green pepper, mushrooms, onions, and other vegetables. SUBTRACT 1 point from your score if you order extra cheese.)*

(a) no cheese with vegetables +3
(b) cheese with vegetables +1
(c) cheese 0
(d) cheese with meat toppings -3
(e) don't eat pizza +2

32. What kind of cookies do you usually eat?

(a) graham crackers or ginger snaps +1
(b) oatmeal -1
(c) sandwich cookies (like Oreos) -2
(d) chocolate coated, chocolate chip, or peanut butter -3
(e) don't eat cookies +3

33. What kind of frozen dessert do you usually eat? *(SUBTRACT 1 point from your score for each topping you use--whipped cream, hot fudge, nuts, etc.)*

(a) gourmet ice cream -3
(b) regular ice cream -1
(c) sorbet, sherbet, or ices +1
(d) frozen yogurt, fat-free ice cream, or ice milk +1
(e) don't eat frozen desserts +3

34. What kind of cake or pastry do you usually eat?

(a) cheesecake, pie, or any microwave cake -3
(b) cake with frosting or filling -2
(c) cake without frosting -1
(d) unfrosted muffin, banana bread, or carrot cake 0
(e) angelfood or fat-free cake +1
(f) don't eat cakes or pastries +3

35. How many times per week does your dinner contain grains, vegetables, or beans, but little or no animal protein (meat, poultry, fish, eggs, milk, or cheese)?

(a) none -1 (c) 3-4 +2
(b) 1-2 +1 (d) 5 or more +3

36. Which of the following salty snacks do you typically eat? *(AVERAGE two or more scores if necessary.)*
(a) potato chips, corn chips, or packaged popcorn -3
(b) reduced-fat potato or tortilla chips -2
(c) salted pretzels -1
(d) unsalted pretzels or baked corn or tortilla chips +1
(e) homemade air-popped popcorn +3
(f) don't eat salty snacks +3

37. What do you usually use to saute vegetables or other foods? *(Vegetable oil includes safflower, corn, canola, olive, sunflower, and soybean.)*
(a) butter or lard -3
(b) more than one tablespoon of margarine or vegetable oil -1
(c) no more than one tablespoon of margarine or vegetable oil 0
(d) no more than one tablespoon of olive oil +1
(e) water or broth +2

38. What kind of cereal do you usually eat?
(a) whole grain (like oatmeal or Shredded Wheat) +3
(b) low fiber (like Cream of Wheat or Corn Flakes) 0
(c) sugary low-fiber (like Frosted Flakes) -1
(d) granola -2

39. With what do you make tuna salad, pasta salad, chicken salad, etc.?
(a) mayonnaise -2
(b) light mayonnaise -1
(c) nonfat mayonnaise 0
(d) low-fat yogurt +2
(e) nonfat yogurt +3

40. What do you typically put on your pasta? *(ADD one point if you also add sauteed vegetables. AVERAGE two or more scores if necessary.)*
(a) tomato sauce +3
(b) tomato sauce with a little Parmesan +3
(c) white clam sauce +1
(d) meat sauce or meat balls -2
(e) Alfredo, pesto, or other creamy sauce -3

Scoring:

+59 to + 116 GREAT! You're a nutrition superstar. Give yourself a big (nonbutter) pat on the back. Continue the good work.

0 to +58 GOOD Pin your Quiz on the nearest wall. Look at areas for improvement.

58 to -1 FAIR Hang in there. Keep a diary of the foods you eat and make daily changes whenever possible.

-117 to -59 ARGHH! Empty your refrigerator and cupboard. It's time to start over.

Source: CSPI Nutrition Quiz, Nutrition Health Action Letter, March 1992, P.O. Box 96611, Washington, D.C. 20090-6611.

Daily Food Diary

Name: ______________________________ Date: ____________

Directions: Keep a record of your daily food intake for one week. Carry this recording sheet with you and note the foods you eat as you eat them. Later, conduct a basic analysis of the nutritional value of your diet. Take note of strengths and weaknesses and use this information to make appropriate changes in your diet.

	Food & Source	Portion Size	Calories	Food Group	Nutrients
Day 1					
Day 2					
Day 3					
Day 4					
Day 5					
Day 6					
Day 7					

Your Eating Habits and Extra Calories

Name: ______________________________ Date: _________

Directions: Think about your eating patterns and habits: What, how much, when, where and why do you eat. For each of these questions, check the answers that best describe your eating patterns and habits.

WHAT do I usually eat?

__ A varied and balanced diet that includes only moderate amounts of fat, and alcoholic beverages.

__ Deep-fat fried and breaded foods.

__ "Extras," such as salad dressings, potato toppings, spreads, sauces and gravies.

__ Sweets and rich desserts such as candies, cakes, pies.

__ Snack foods high in fat and sodium, such as chips and other "munchies."

__ Cocktails, wine and beer.

HOW MUCH do I usually eat?

__ A single, small serving.

__ A large serving.

__ Two servings or more.

WHEN do I usually eat?

__ At mealtime only.

__ While preparing meals or clearing the table.

__ While watching TV or participating in other activities.

__ At coffee break.

__ Anytime.

WHERE do I usually eat?

__ At the kitchen or dining room table.

__ At restaurants or fast food places.

__ In front of the TV or while reading.

__ Wherever I happen to be when I'm "hungry."

WHY do I usually eat?

__ It's time to eat.

__ I'm "starved."

__ Foods look tempting.

__ Everyone else is eating.

__ Food will get thrown away if I don't eat it.

__ I'm bored or frustrated.

Analysis: Look at the boxes you checked for "what" and "how much" you eat. Do they provide any clues to where your extra calories are coming from? Your answers to "when, where, and why" you eat are important too. They often affect **what** and **how much** you eat.

Can you identify some habits that may be due for a change? Try to think of ways to modify "problem" habits. If, for example, you often nibble while doing other things, make an effort to plan your meals and snacks ahead of time. For eating at home, make a rule to eat only while sitting at the kitchen or dining room table. If candy bars from the vending machine at your office coffee break are a problem, substitute a low-calorie snack brought from home. If you often eat because you're bored or frustrated think of other activities to get your mind off food-jog, call a friend, or walk the dog.

Why Do You Eat? Inventory

Name: ________________________________ Date: __________

Directions: Here are some statements made by people to describe what they get out of eating. How *often* do you feel this way about eating? Circle one number for each statement. *Important*: Answer every question.

Response Scale:	5 Always	4 Frequently	3 Occasionally	2 Seldom	1 Never

A. I eat to keep myself from slowing down.
Always 5 4 3 2 1 Never

B. Handling food is part of the enjoyment of eating.
Always 5 4 3 2 1 Never

C. Eating is pleasant and relaxing.
Always 5 4 3 2 1 Never

D. When I feel angry about something, I eat.
Always 5 4 3 2 1 Never

E. When I run out of my favorite foods I find it almost unbearable until I can get more.
Always 5 4 3 2 1 Never

F. I eat automatically without even being aware of it.
Always 5 4 3 2 1 Never

G. I eat to stimulate me, perk myself up.
Always 5 4 3 2 1 Never

H. Part of the enjoyment of eating comes from the steps I take to prepare the food.
Always 5 4 3 2 1 Never

I. I find eating pleasurable.
Always 5 4 3 2 1 Never

J. When I feel uncomfortable or upset about something, I eat.
Always 5 4 3 2 1 Never

K. I am very much aware of the fact when I am not eating.
Always 5 4 3 2 1 Never

L. I eat without realizing what I am doing.
Always 5 4 3 2 1 Never

M. I eat to give me a "lift."
Always 5 4 3 2 1 Never

O. I want food most when I am comfortable and relaxed.
Always 5 4 3 2 1 Never

P. When I feel "blue" or want to take my mind off cares and worries, I eat.
Always 5 4 3 2 1 Never

Q. I get a real gnawing hunger for food when I haven's eaten for a while.
Always 5 4 3 2 1 Never

R. I've found food in my mouth and didn't remember putting it there.
Always 5 4 3 2 1 Never

Scoring:

1. Enter the numbers you have circled to the test questions in the following spaces, putting the number you circled to question A over line A, to question B over line B, and so on.
2. Total the three scores on each line to get your totals. For example, the sum of your scores over lines A, G, and M gives you your score on "Stimulation"; lines B, H, and N give you the score on "Handling," and so on.

							Totals
____	+	____	+	____	=		____________
A		G		M			Stimulation
____	+	____	+	____	=		____________
B		H		N			Handling
____	+	____	+	____	=		____________
C		I		O			Pleasurable relaxation
____	+	____	+	____	=		____________
D		J		P			Crutch: tension reduction
____	+	____	+	____	=		____________
E		K		Q			Craving: psychological addiction
____	+	____	+	____	=		____________
F		L		R			Habit

Scores can vary from 3 to 15. Any score 11 and above is high; any score 7 and below is low.

Interpretation: The six factors measured by this instrument describe one or another way of experiencing or managing certain kinds of feelings. Three of these feeling states represent the positive feelings people get from eating: (1) a sense of increased energy or *stimulation*; (2) the satisfaction of *handling* or manipulating things; and (3) the enhancing of *pleasurable feelings* by reducing the state of tension or feelings of anxiety, anger, and shame, for example. The fifth is a complex pattern of increasing and decreasing "craving" for eating that represents a *psychological addiction* to food. The sixth, *habit*, is eating that occurs in an absence of feeling--purely automatic eating.

A score of 11 or above on any factor indicates that this factor is an important source of satisfaction for you. The higher your score (15 is the highest), the more important a particular factor is in your eating and the more useful the discussion of that factor can be in your attempt to cut down on eating.

If you do not score high on any of the six factors, chances are that you are not an excessive eater. If so, cutting down calories should be easy.

If you score high on several categories, you apparently get several kinds of satisfaction from eating and will have to find several solutions. Certain combinations of scores may indicate that reducing food intake will be especially difficult. Those who score high on both factor 4 and factor 5, "reduction of negative feelings and craving," may have a hard time cutting down on caloric intake. However, there are ways to do it; many excessive eaters represented by this combination have been able to cut down on caloric intake.

Others who score high on factors 4 and 5 may find it useful to change their patterns of eating and cut down at the same time. They can try to eat foods that are lower in calories such as carrots, fresh fruits, Ry-Crisp, or to substitute exercise and other physical activities for eating. After several months of trying this solution, they may find it easier to develop a habit pattern of low-calorie intake.

You must make a decision to cut down caloric intake either by (1) substituting appropriate volumes of less fattening foods for the high-calorie foods currently in your diet; or (2) reducing or eliminating excess calorie food (like junk food) from your diet without the substitution of low-calorie foods.

Source: Walter Sorochan, Promoting Your Health. New York: John Wiley & Sons, 1981, pp. 175-79. Adapted from Smoker's Self-Testing Kit, PHS Publication No. 1904, 1969, developed by Daniel Horn, Director of the National Clearinghouse for Smoking and Health of the Public Health Service and members of the Clearinghouse staff.

Do You Have An Eating Disorder?

Name: ______________________ Date: __________

Directions: Answer yes or no to the following questions.

___ 1. Are you intensely afraid of becoming fat?

___ 2. Do you feel fat even though others say you are thin and emaciated?

___ 3. Do you like to shop for food and cook for others but prefer not to eat the meals you make?

___ 4. Do you have eating rituals (e.g., cutting food into tiny bites, eating only certain foods in a particular order or at a particular time of day)?

___ 5. Have you lost 25 percent or more of your minimum body weight through diets and fasts?

___ 6. When you feel hungry, do you usually refrain from eating?

___ 7. If you are a female of childbearing age, have you stopped menstruating?

___ 8. Do you often experience cold hands and feet, dry skin, or cracked fingernails?

___ 9. Do you have a covering of fuzzy hair over your body?

___ 10. Do you often feel depressed, angry, guilty, or inadequate?

___ 11. When people express concern about your low weight, do you deny that anything is wrong?

___ 12. Do you often exercise strenuously or for long periods of time even when you feel tired or sick?

___ 13. Have you ever eaten a large amount of food and then fasted, forced yourself to vomit, or used laxatives, diuretics, or enemas to purge yourself?

___ 14. Are you frequently on a rigid diet?

___ 15. Do you regularly experience stomachaches or constipation?

___ 16. Do you eat large quantities of food in a short period of time, usually high-calorie foods that can be easily digested (e.g., bread, pasta, cake, cookies, ice-cream, or mashed potatoes)?

___ 17. Do you eat in secret, hide food, or lie about your eating?

___ 18. Have you ever stolen food or money to buy food so that you could start or continue a binge?

___ 19. Do you feel guilty and remorseful about your eating behavior?

___ 20. Do you start eating even when you are not hungry?

___ 21. Is it hard for you to stop eating even when you want to?

___ 22. Do you eat to escape problems, to relax, or to have fun?

___ 23. After finishing a meal, do you worry about making it to the next meal without getting hungry in between?

___ 24. Have others expressed concern about your obsession with food?

___ 25. Do you worry that your eating behavior is abnormal?

___ 26. Do you fall asleep after eating?

___ 27. Do you regularly fast, use laxatives or diet pill, induce vomiting, or exercise excessively to avoid gaining weight?

___ 28. Does your weight fluctuate 10 pounds or more between alternate periods of bingeing and purging?

___ 29. Are your neck glands swollen?

___ 30. Do you have scars on the backs of your hands from forced vomiting?

Scoring: Five or more "yes" answers within any of the following three groups of questions strongly suggest the presence of an eating disorder: questions 1-15, anorexia nervosa; questions 14-26, compulsive eating; questions 12-30, bulimia. Which behaviors are most problematic for you? What can you do to ensure that you minimize the damage you may have already caused to your body and psyche, and to prevent any further damage?

Source: Adapted from Barbara Yoder, The Recovery Resource Book. New York: Simon and Schuster, 1990 p. 159.

Check Your Cholesterol and Heart Disease I.Q.

Directions

Are you cholesterol smart? Test your knowledge about high blood cholesterol with the following questions. Circle each true or false.

T F 1. High blood cholesterol is one of the risk factors for heart disease that you can do something about.

T F 2. To lower your blood cholesterol level you must stop eating meat altogether.

T F 3. Any blood cholesterol level below 240 mg/dL is desirable for adults.

T F 4. Fish oil supplements are recommended to lower blood cholesterol.

T F 5. To lower your blood cholesterol level you should eat less saturated fat, total fat, and cholesterol, and lose weight if you are overweight.

T F 6. Saturated fats raise your blood cholesterol level more than anything else in your diet.

T F 7. All vegetable oils help lower blood cholesterol levels.

T F 8. Lowering blood cholesterol levels can help people who have already had a heart attack.

T F 9. All children need to have their blood cholesterol levels checked.

T F 10. Women don't need to worry about high blood cholesterol and heart disease.

T F 11. Reading food labels can help you eat the heart healthy way.

Scoring

Compare your responses with these answers to the Cholesterol and Heart Disease I.Q. Quiz:

1. True.
High blood cholesterol is one of the risk factors for heart disease that a person can do something about. High blood pressure, cigarette smoking, diabetes, overweight, and physical inactivity are the others.

2. False.
Although some red meat is high in saturated fat and cholesterol, which can raise your blood cholesterol, you do not need to stop eating it or any other single food. Red meat is an important source of protein, iron, and other vitamins and minerals. You should, however, cut back on the amount of saturated fat and cholesterol that you eat. One way to do this is by choosing lean cuts of meat with the fat trimmed. Another way is to watch your portion sizes and eat no more than 6 ounces of meat a day. Six ounces is about the size of two decks of playing cards.

3. False.
A total blood cholesterol level of under 200 mg/dL is desirable and usually puts you at a lower risk for heart disease. A blood cholesterol level of 240 mg/dL is high and increases your risk of heart disease. If your cholesterol level is high, your doctor will want to check your level of LDL-cholesterol ("bad" cholesterol). A HIGH level of LDL-cholesterol increases your risk of heart disease, as does a LOW level of HDL-cholesterol ("good" cholesterol). An HDL-cholesterol level below 35 mg/dL is considered a risk factor for heart disease. A total cholesterol level of 200 239 mg/dL is considered borderline-high and usually increases your risk for heart disease. All adults 20 years of age or older should have their blood cholesterol level checked at least once every 5 years.

4. False.
Fish oils are a source of omega-3 fatty acids, which are a type of polyunsaturated fat. Fish oil supplements generally do not reduce blood cholesterol levels. Also, the effect of the long-term use of fish oil supplements is not known. However, fish is a good food choice because it is low in saturated fat.

5. True.
Eating less fat, especially saturated fat, and cholesterol can lower your blood cholesterol level. Generally your blood cholesterol level should begin to drop a few weeks after you start on a cholesterol-lowering diet. How much your level drops depends on the amounts of saturated fat and cholesterol you used to eat, how high your blood cholesterol is, how much weight you lose if you are overweight, and how your body responds to the changes you make. Over time, you may reduce your blood cholesterol level by 10-50 mg/dL or even more.

6. True.
Saturated fats raise your blood cholesterol level more than anything else. So, the best way to reduce your cholesterol level is to cut back on the amount of saturated fats that you eat. These fats are found in largest amounts in animal products such as butter, cheese, whole milk, ice cream, cream, and fatty meats. They are also found in some vegetable oils--coconut, palm, and palm kernel oils.

7. False.
Most vegetable oils--canola, corn, olive, safflower, soybean, and sunflower oils--contain mostly monounsaturated and polyunsaturated fats, which help lower blood cholesterol when used in place of saturated fats. However, a few vegetable oils– coconut, palm, and palm kernel oils -contain more saturated fat than unsaturated fat. A special kind of fat, called "trans fat," is formed when vegetable oil is hardened to become margarine or shortening, through a process called "hydrogenation." The harder the margarine or shortening, the more likely it is to contain more trans fat. Choose margarine containing liquid vegetable oil as the first ingredient. Just be sure to limit the total amount of any fats or oils, since even those that are unsaturated are rich sources of calories.

8. True.
People who have had one heart attack are at much higher risk for a second attack. Reducing blood cholesterol levels can greatly slow down (and, in some people, even reverse) the buildup of cholesterol and fat in the wall of the coronary arteries and significantly reduce the chances of a second heart attack. If you have had a heart attack or have coronary disease, your LDL level should be around 100 mg/dL which is even lower than the recommended level of less than 130 mg/dL for the general population.

9. False.
Children from "high risk" families, in which a parent has high blood cholesterol (240 mg/dL or above) or in which a parent or grandparent has had heart disease at an early age (at 55 years or younger), should have their cholesterol levels tested. If a child from such a family has a cholesterol level that is high, it should be lowered under medical supervision, primarily with diet, to reduce the risk of developing heart disease as an adult. For most children, who are not from high-risk families, the best way to reduce the risk of adult heart disease is to follow a low saturated fat, low cholesterol eating pattern. All children over the age of 2 years and all adults should adopt a heart healthy eating pattern as a principal way of reducing coronary heart disease.

10. False.
Blood cholesterol levels in both men and women begin to go up around age 20. Women before menopause have levels that are lower than men of the same age. After menopause, a women's LDL-cholesterol level goes up-and so her risk for heart disease increases. For both men and women, heart disease is the number one cause of death.

11. True.
Food labels have been changed. Look on the nutrition label for the amount of saturated fat, total fat, cholesterol, and total calories in a serving of the product. Use this information to compare similar products. Also, look for the list of ingredients. Here, the ingredient in the greatest amount is first and the ingredient in the least amount is last. So to choose foods low in saturated fat or total fat, go easy on products that list fats or oil first, or that list many fat and oil ingredients.

Source: National Cholesterol Education Program, National Heart, Lung, and Blood Institute, U.S. Department of Health and Human Services, National Institutes of Health

Your Exercise Contract

Name: ______________________________________ Date: ____________

Directions: Make a written agreement with yourself about exercise. Set specific goals in Section 1 for increasing your energy and specific goals in Section 2 for increasing activity. Start slowly. Even a 100 calorie expenditure per day produces a weight loss of ten to twelve pounds in one year.

Remember to motivate yourself through a reward system in Section 3. List specific daily and weekly rewards for meeting your exercise goals. Self-payments may range from eating special foods to treating yourself to a night out. Choose rewards that are not destructive to your overall fitness program.

During this week _____________ 19______, I hereby agree to work as hard as possible at achieving the following:

1. Physical activity goals for increasing my energy use during occupational time:

   A. I will park my car or leave public transportation and walk ___ additional minutes per day.

   B. I will spend ___ minutes daily standing instead of sitting while I work.

   C. I will walk up ___ flights of stairs each work day.

   D. I will walk around my work area ___ minutes every day.

   E. I will spend ___ minutes during each coffee break standing instead of sitting.

   F. I will spend ___ minutes during each lunch break walking outside in the open air.

2. Physical activity goals for increasing my energy use during recreational time:

   A. I will spend ___ minutes daily doing stretching activities to increase my flexibility.

   B. I will spend ___ minutes at least three times per week doing aerobic activities to improve my endurance.

   C. I will spend ___ minutes at least three times per week doing strength activities.

   D. I will spend ___ minutes Saturday and Sunday in active recreational activities.

3. My rewards and consequences:

   A. I will reward myself daily with one of the following pleasures when I achieve my daily goals in increased activity:

1. ______________________________ 4. ______________________________

2. ______________________________ 5. ______________________________

3. ______________________________ 6. ______________________________

B. When I do *not* make my daily goals I agree to do the following:

1. ______________________ 2. ______________________

C. I will reward myself every week with one of the following pleasures when I achieve my weekly exercise goals:

1. ______________________ 4. ______________________

2. ______________________ 5. ______________________

3. ______________________ 6. ______________________

D. When I do *not* make my weekly goals I agree to do the following:

1. ______________________ 2. ______________________

I now agree to the above contract and with the goals and consequences. I also agree to follow this contract until my goals are reached.

Signed ______________________ Date ______________________

Witnessed ______________________

Source: Jerrold S. Greenberg/George B. Dintiman, Exploring Health. Englewood Cliffs, NJ: Prentice Hall, p. 225.

How Much Do I Move?

Name: ______________________________________ Date: ___________

Directions: We often have an unrealistic perception of how much we actively move. Be as honest as possible when assessing the amount that you move during the average day. If it is different on weekends, fill out for days during the week and weekend separately.

1. Types of movement. Check off those in which you participate.

Walking	___	Hiking	___
Climbing	___	Jogging/Running	___
Lifting weights	___	Team sports	___
Tennis	___	Dancing	___
Lovemaking	___	Bicycling	___
Swimming	___	Aerobics	___
Step climbing	___	Yoga	___
Jumping rope	___	Skiing	___
Physical labor	___	Ice skating	___
Other	___		

2. Time spent moving or exercising:

   Daily _______________ minutes Weekend _______________

   Weekly _______________ Min./Hrs.

   Monthly _______________ Min./Hrs.

3. Record the amount of time spent exercising during the month. _______

4. Do you spend as much time moving as you would like? _______________

5. If not, in what types of activity would you like to participate?

   ____

   ____

   ____

6. What small change will you make toward improving your degree of movement?

   ____

   ____

7. What are you going to do today to implement the small change? _____

   ____

   ____

8. What will you do tomorrow? ______________________________

____

____

9. What will you do this weekend? ____________________________

____

____

10. What will you do this month? _____________________________

____

____

11. What reward will you give yourself for meeting your objective? _____

____

____

Check Your Physical Activity & Heart Disease I.Q.

Directions

Test how much you know about how physical activity affects your heart. Mark each statement true or false.

True False 1. Regular physical activity can reduce your chances of getting heart disease.

True False 2. Most people get enough physical activity from their normal daily routine.

True False 3. You don't have to train like a marathon runner to become more physically fit.

True False 4. Exercise programs do not require a lot of time to be very effective.

True False 5. People who need to lose some weight are the only ones who will benefit from regular physical activity.

True False 6. All exercises give you the same benefits.

True False 7. The older you are, the less active you need to be.

True False 8. It doesn't take a lot of money or expensive equipment to become physically fit.

True False 9. There are many risks and injuries that can occur with exercise.

True False 10. You should consult a doctor before starting a physical activity program.

True False 11. People who have had a heart attack should not start any physical activity program.

True False 12. To help stay physically active, include a variety of activities.

Scoring

Compare your responses with the following answers to the Check Your Physical Activity and Heart Disease I.Q. Quiz

1. True.

Heart disease is almost twice as likely to develop in inactive people. Being physically inactive is a risk factor for heart disease along with cigarette smoking, high blood pressure, high blood cholesterol, and being overweight. The more risk factors you have, the greater your chance for heart disease. Regular physical activity (even mild to moderate exercise) can reduce this risk.

2. False.
Most Americans are very busy but not very active. Every American adult should make a habit of getting 30 minutes of low to moderate levels of physical activity daily. This includes walking, gardening, and walking up stairs. If you are inactive now, begin by doing a few minutes of activity each day. If you only do some activity every once in a while, try to work something into your routine everyday.

3. True.
Low- to moderate-intensity activities, such as pleasure walking, stair climbing, yardwork, housework, dancing, and home exercises can have both short- and long-term benefits. If you are inactive, the key is to get started. One great way is to take a walk for 10 to 15 minutes during your lunch break, or take your dog for a walk every day. At least 30 minutes of physical activity everyday can help improve your heart health.

4. True.
It takes only a few minutes a day to become more physically active. If you don t have 30 minutes in your schedule for an exercise break, try to find two 15-minute periods or even three 10-minute periods. These exercise breaks will soon become a habit you can't live without.

5. False.
People who are physically active experience many positive benefits. Regular physical activity gives you more energy, reduces stress, and helps you to sleep better. It helps to lower high blood pressure and improves blood cholesterol levels. Physical activity helps to tone your muscles, burns off calories to help you lose extra pounds or stay at your desirable weight, and helps control your appetite. It can also increase muscle strength, help your heart and lungs work more efficiently, and let you enjoy your life more fully.

6. False.
Low-intensity activities--if performed daily--can have some long-term health benefits and can lower your riskof heart disease. Regular, brisk, and sustained exercise for at least 30 minutes, three to four times a week, such as brisk walking, jogging, or swimming, is necessary to improve the efficiency of your heart and lungs and burn off extra calories. These activities are called aerobic--meaning the body uses oxygen to produce the energy needed for the activity. Other activities, depending on the type, may give you other benefits such as increased flexibility or muscle strength.

7. False.
Although we tend to become less active with age, physical activity is still important. In fact, regular physical activity in older persons increases their capacity to do everyday activities. In general, middle-aged and older people benefit from regular physical activity just as young people do. What is important, at any age, is tailoring the activity program to your own fitness level.

8. True.
Many activities require little or no equipment. For example, brisk walking only requires a comfortable pair of walking shoes. Many communities offer free or inexpensive recreation facilities and physical activity classes. Check your shopping malls, as many of them are open early and late for people who do not wish to walk alone, in the dark, or in bad weather.

9. False.
The most common risk in exercising is injury to the muscles and joints. Such injuries are usually caused by exercising too hard for too long, particularly if a person has been inactive. To avoid injuries, try to build up your level of activity gradually, listen to your body for warning pains, be aware of possible signs of heart problems (such as pain or pressure in the left or mid-chest area, left neck, shoulder, or arm during or just after exercising, or sudden light-headedness, cold sweat, pallor, or fainting), and be prepared for special weather conditions.

10. True.
You should ask your doctor before you start (or greatly increase) your physical activity if you have a medical condition such as high blood pressure, have pains or pressure in the chest and shoulder, feel dizzy or faint, get breathless after mild exertion, are middle-aged or older and have not been physically active, or plan a vigorous activity program. If none of these apply, start slow and get moving.

11. False.
Regular, physical activity can help reduce your risk of having another heart attack. People who include regular physical activity in their lives after a heart attack improve their chances of survival and can improve how they feel and look. If you have had a heart attack, consult your doctor to be sure you are following a safe and effective exercise program that will help prevent heart pain and further damage from overexertion.

12. True.
Pick several different activities that you like doing. You will be more likely to stay with it. Plan short-term and long-term goals. Keep a record of your progress, and check it regularly to see the progress you have made. Get your family and friends to join in. They can help keep you going.

Source : NHLBI Obesity Education Initiative, National Heart, Lung, and Blood Institute, National Institutes of Health, Originally Printed 1995, Reprinted August 1996

The Muscle Hustle: Test Your Exercise I.Q.

Directions

Circle "True" or "False" for each statement.

True False 1. Be wary of exercise devices that promise total fitness "in just three minutes a day."

True False 2. Even when they are relaxing, people who exercise regularly burn more calories than inactive people.

True False 3. The total price of an exercise machine that's advertised at "4 easy payments of $50" is about $200.

True False 4. Weight lifting has no health benefit.

True False 5. Sit-ups and ab crunches are the best way to burn fat off the stomach.

True False 6. Cross-training is the best route to overall fitness.

True False 7. It's best to buy exercise equipment that comes with a "money-back guarantee."

True False 8. No exercise device can help you spot reduce.

True False 9. Before-and-after claims in ads for exercise devices may be misleading.

Scoring

1. TRUE. Real fitness requires regular activity, sensible eating and a healthy lifestyle. Exercise need not be grueling, but there are no "three minute a day" shortcuts to better flexibility, improved muscular strength, enhanced physical endurance, or improved cardiovascular or respiratory efficiency—or weight loss.

2. TRUE. Everyone burns calories while they're exercising. But one of the great benefits of an active lifestyle is that it can boost your metabolism even when you're at rest.

3. FALSE. Shipping charges, postage, handling, delivery, or other hidden fees can add on to the cost of exercise equipment. Whether you order by phone or buy at a retail store, find out the real cost before making a purchase.

4. FALSE. Strength training isn't just for the "body beautiful" types. Lean muscle burns more calories than flab. Sensible weight training helps maintain muscle tone and endurance.

5. FALSE. The most common cause of a "beer belly" is fat—not weak muscles. Sit-ups may help tone the abs, but only a sensible diet combined with regular exercise can turn a "beer belly" into a "six pack stomach."

6. TRUE. Cross-training—a regular program combining different types of activity—is your best route to fitness. A combination of your favorite activities—walking, swimming, biking, dancing—can help you shape up while avoiding the boredom and burnout of one kind of exercise.

7. TRUE. But get the facts first. Not all "money-back guarantees" are the same. How long do you have to return the equipment? If you order through the mail, how much will it cost to return it? Who pays for repairs?

8. TRUE. No exercise device can burn fat off a particular part of your body. The reason: Everything you eat has calories, and everything you do uses calories. Your weight depends on the number of calories you eat and use each day. Increasing your daily physical activity will burn extra calories.

9. TRUE. Before-and-after pictures can be eye-catching, but they may not always tell the whole story. Regular exercise is an important ingredient in moving from plump to "pumped," but diet plays a key part, too.

Source: FTC Briefs, June 1997, Consumer Response Center, Federal Trade Commission, 600 Pennsylvania Ave, NW, Washington, DC

Marijuana Attitudes

Name: ______________________________________ Date: ____________

Directions: What do you think? How strongly do you feel about the following items? Place each letter in a numbered box to rank order the lettered items according to your depth of feeling about each statement.

A. The smoking of pot in public places.
B. People getting long prison sentences for possession of marijuana.
C. Organizations that advocate legalization of marijuana.
D. Merchants and magazines that specialize in "head" products.
E. Younger people you know and care about using marijuana.
F. Friends who make a habit of turning on their nondrug-using friends.

Strongest feeling — Weakest feeling

1	2	3	4	5	6

What values are reflected by your feelings? Do you need to examine some issues further in order to render values to choices regarding marijuana? What ones?

Source: Corry, et al., Drugs: Facts, Alternatives and Decisions. New York: Wadsworth, 1985.

Why People Use Drugs

Name: ______________________________ Date: __________

Directions: What Are Your Psychoactive Drug Use Motives? Rank order the following questions according to the ones most appropriate for you (if you have never used any psychoactive drugs, try to imagine what your answers might be).

I use drugs because

___ 1. Drugs allow me to escape from an annoying world.

___ 2. Drugs help me to achieve an altered state of consciousness.

___ 3. Drugs allow me to hang around some interesting people.

___ 4. I'm not afraid of life when I'm using drugs.

___ 5. Drugs are a part of my culture; they're just natural to use.

___ 6. Drug use allows me to feel good about myself.

___ 7. Drugs help me to be a more spiritual person.

___ 8. Drugs are my way of protesting the ugliness of the world.

___ 9. My drug use is a social protest against the system.

___ 10. Drugs are the only thing of interest about me or my life.

___ 11. Drugs are a source of enjoyment; they're just playthings.

___ 12. My drugs are really food (e.g., beer, wine, tea or coffee).

___ 13. My friends would think less of me if I didn't use drugs.

___ 14. I need drugs to get me through a day.

___ 15. Drugs help me to experience the world in a very special way, and I can't duplicate this without drugs.

___ 16. Drugs are a source of relief from tension.

___ 17. Drugs allow me to be more social.

___ 18.*______________________________

___ 19.*______________________________

___ 20.*______________________________

* (Add your own)

Source: Corry et al., Drugs: Facts, Alternatives and Decision. New York: Wadsworth, 1985.

Do You Have A Drug Problem?

Name: ______________________________ Date: ____________

Directions: Answer the following questions by placing a check next to the appropriate boxes.

1. Which of the following have you tried more than once outside the direct care of a physician? (Score 2 points for each box checked)
   [ ] caffeine
   [ ] cannabis (hashish, marijuana)
   [ ] cocaine powder
   [ ] crack
   [ ] PCP (angel dust)
   [ ] heroin, methadone, morphine
   [ ] LSD
   [ ] amphetamines
   [ ] barbiturates
   [ ] benzodiazapines (Valium and Librium)

2. How often do you use some form of psychoactive drug?
   [ ] daily or almost daily (16 points)
   [ ] more often than once a week but less than daily (8 points)
   [ ] about once a week (4 points)
   [ ] about once a month (2 points)
   [ ] rarely if ever (1 point)

3. How would you feel if you did not use any psychoactive drug for more than three days?
   [ ] I would be very nervous and upset and have an uncontrollable urge to find a drug to use. (16 points)
   [ ] I would want to use a drug very much but could definitely control myself. (8 points)
   [ ] I would think quite a bit about using a drug. (4 points)
   [ ] I would think a little about using a drug. (2 points)
   [ ] I wouldn't notice that I hadn't used it. (1 point)

4. Which of the following have you recently experienced that accompanied your use of drugs? (Score 3 points for each box checked)
   [ ] missing work or school
   [ ] fighting with family or friends
   [ ] becoming belligerent, insulting, or fighting
   [ ] chest pains
   [ ] difficulty breathing
   [ ] feelings of dizziness, nausea, or vertigo

5. Which of the following have you experienced recently? (Score 2 points for each box checked.)
   [ ] withdrawal symptoms when drug use has been delayed
   [ ] an ability to take increased doses of a drug
   [ ] a need to take an increased dose of a drug to get a desired effect
   [ ] no effect from a drug that used to get you high

[ ] the use of a drug at the same time every day
[ ] losing track of how many times you have used a drug or how much you have taken
[ ] using more than one drug during the same time period.

Scoring: Total the points as indicated with each question.

Interpretation:

Score	Label	Danger Rating
2-5	Nonuser	x
6-19	Experimenter	xx
20-35	Moderate user	xxxxx
36-50	Heavy user	xxxxxxxxx
51-90	Problem user	xxxxxxxxxxxx-see a counselor *now*

Source: Joan Luckman, Your Health!. Englewood Cliffs, NJ: Prentice Hall, 1990.

Evaluating Drug Use Presentation in Movies

Name: ______________________________ Date: ________

Directions: For the film being observed, respond to the following statements by circling one of the following choices located under each statement.

SA = Strongly Agree
A = Agree
U = Undecided
D = Disagree
SD = Strongly disagree
NA = Not Applicable (drug-related scenes not in film)

Title of Film ______________________________

Number of drug use scenes in the film ____

Generally the scene in the film or movie:

1. Encourages or condones the use of mood modifying substances.
   SA A U D SD NA
2. Does not show the negative effects of using mood modifying substances.
   SA A U D SD NA
3. Promotes use of mood modifying substances as a solution to boredom.
   SA A U D SD NA
4. Associates the use of mood modifying substances with fun or pleasure.
   SA A U D SD NA
5. Encourages the use of mood modifying substances as a problem-solving behavior.
   SA A U D SD NA
6. Suggests that use of mood modifying substances is a "norm" (in other words, "everyone is doing it!").
   SA A U D SD NA
7. Portrays people who abstain from using mood modifying substances as immature, not adult, or "nerds."
   SA A U D SD NA
8. Shows an easy solution to the results of misuse or abuse of mood modifying substances.
   SA A U D SD NA
9. Portrays the hero or heroine as one who uses mood modifying substances.
   SA A U D SD NA
10. Portrays the use of mood modifying substances as a means of enhancing performance (intellectual, physical, spiritual, etc.).
   SA A U D SD NA

Scoring and Interpretation:

Step I: Scoring: Use the following method of scoring your responses:

[SA]	Strongly Agree	= 5 points
[A]	Agree	= 4 points
[U]	Undecided	= 3 points
[D]	Disagree	= 2 points
[SD]	Strongly Disagree	= 1 point
[NA]	Not Applicable	= 0 points

Step II: Add your points as follows:

Statement 1:	______	Points	Statement 6:	______	Points
+			+		
Statement 2:	______	Points	Statement 7:	______	Points
+			+		
Statement 3:	______	Points	Statement 8:	______	Points
+			+		
Statement 4:	______	Points	Statement 9:	______	Points
+			+		
Statement 5:	______	Points	Statement 10:	______	Points
+			=		
			Total Points	______	

Step III: After you have added up the total points, place an "X" on the appropriate point on the following line that best represents your total points. Once you've placed the "X" that represents the total points, you can easily see the film's position regarding drug use.

"Anti" Drug Use Position | "Pro" Drug Use Position

< ----------|----------|----------|---------->

10 20 30 40 50

Step IV: Comments regarding analysis of movie (e.g., what kind of closure was reached?).

Passive Smoking

Name: ______________________________ Date: __________

Directions: Answer the following questions to assess your attitudes toward and exposure to passive smoke. Describe your thoughts, feelings, or behavior in response to each question.

1. How many people in your home, apartment, or dorm room smoke?

____

____

2. Does your employer provide separate work/break areas for smokers and nonsmokers?

____

____

3. Are smokers in your home or work environment considerate of nonsmokers (If you smoke, are you considerate of nonsmokers)?

____

____

4. When I go to a restaurant with smokers, (or with nonsmokers and you are a smoker), I:

____

____

5. When I travel in a car with smokers (or with nonsmokers and you are a smoker), I:

____

____

6. The things that bother me most about being around smokers are:

____

____

Interpretation: Perhaps use these questions to initiate discussion with family, friends, employers, or co-workers about the effects of passive smoking and the rights of non-smokers.

Is Someone You Know an Inhalant Abuser?

Directions

Indicate which symptoms or behaviors seem to be present:

Yes	No	Unusual breath odor or chemical odor on clothing.
Yes	No	Slurred or disoriented speech.
Yes	No	Drunk, dazed, or dizzy appearance.
Yes	No	Signs of paint or other products where they wouldn't normally be, such as on the face or fingers.
Yes	No	Red or runny eyes or nose.
Yes	No	Spots and/or sores around the mouth.
Yes	No	Nausea and/or loss of appetite.
Yes	No	Anxiety, excitability, irritability, or restlessness.
Yes	No	Sitting with a pen or marker near nose.
Yes	No	Constantly smelling clothing sleeves.
Yes	No	Hiding rags, clothes, or empty containers of the potentially abused products in closets and other places.

Scoring

If some or all these symptoms or behaviors are evident, then the person may be an inhalant abuser. There is no typical profile of an inhalant abuser. Victims are represented by both sexes and all socioeconomic groups throughout the U.S.

Source: Developed from information provided by A Parent's Guide to Preventing Inhalant Abuse, U.S. Consumer Product Safety Commission

Drinking Related Internal-External Locus of Control Scale

Directions

These are questions to find out the way in which certain important events in our society affect different people. Each item consists of a pair of alternatives lettered a or b. Please select the one statement of each pair (and only one) which you more strongly believe to be the case as far as you are concerned. Be sure to select the one you actually believe to be more true rather than the one you would like to be true. This is a measure of personal belief: obviously there are no right or wrong answers.

Please answer these items carefully but do not spend too much time on any one item. Be sure to find an answer for every choice. Find the number of the item and circle either letter a or b, whichever one you choose to be the one more true.

In some instances you may discover that you believe both statements or neither one. In such cases, be sure to select the one you more strongly believe to be the case as far as you're concerned. Also try to respond to each item independently when making your choice; do not be influenced by your previous choices.

1. a. One of the major reasons why people drink is because they cannot handle their problems.

   b. People drink because circumstances force them to.

2. a. The idea that men or women are driven to drink by their spouses is nonsense.

   b. Most people do not realize that drinking problems are influenced by accidental happenings.

3. a. I feel so helpless in some situations that I need a drink.

   b. Abstinence is just a matter of deciding that I no longer want to drink.

4. a. I have the strength to withstand pressures at work.

   b. Trouble at work or home drives me to drink.

5. a. Without the right breaks one cannot stay sober.

   b. Alcoholics who are not successful in curbing their drinking often have not taken advantage of help that is available.

6. a. There is no such thing as an irresistable temptation to drink.

   b. Many times there are circumstances that force you to drink.

7. a. I get so upset over small arguments, that they cause me to drink.

   b. I can usually handle arguments without taking a drink.

8. a. Successfully licking alcoholism is a matter of hard work, luck has little to do with it.

b. Staying sober depends mainly on things going right for you.

9. a. When I see a bottle, I cannot resist taking a drink.

   b. It is no more difficult for me to resist drinking when I am near a bottle than when I am not.

10. a. The average person has an influence on whether he drinks or not.

    b. Oftentimes, other people drive one to drink.

11. a. When I am at a party where others are drinking, I can avoid taking a drink.

    b. It is impossible for me to resist drinking if I am at a party where others are drinking.

12. a. Those who are successful in quitting drinking are the ones who are just plain lucky.

    b. Quitting drinking depends upon lots of effort and hard work (luck has little or nothing to do with it.)

13. a. I feel powerless to prevent myself from drinking when I am anxious or unhappy.

    b. If I really wanted to, I could stop drinking.

14. a. It is easy for me to have a good time when I am sober.

    b. I cannot feel good unless I am drinking.

15. a. As far as drinking is concerned, most of us are victims of forces we can neither understand or control.

    b. By taking an active part in our treatment programs, we can control our drinking.

16. a. I have control over my drinking behavior.

    b. I feel completely helpless when it comes to resisting a drink.

17. a. If people want to badly enough, they can change their drinking behavior.

    b. It is impossible for some people to ever stop drinking.

18. a. With enough effort we can lick our drinking.

    b. It is difficult for alcoholics to have much control over their drinking.

19. a. If someone offers me a drink, I cannot refuse him.

    b. I have the strength to refuse a drink.

20. a. Sometimes I cannot understand how people can control their drinking.

b. There is a direct connection between how hard people try and how successful they are in stopping their drinking.

21. a. I can overcome my urge to drink.

b. Once I start to drink I can't stop.

22. a. Drink isn't necessary in order to solve my problems.

b. I just cannot handle my problems unless I take a drink first.

23. a. Most of the time I can't understand why I continue drinking.

b. In the long run, I an responsible for my drinking problems

24. a. If I make up my mind, I can stop drinking.

b. I have no will power when it comes to drinking.

25. a. Drinking is my favorite form of entertainment.

b. It wouldn't bother me if I could never have another drink.

Scoring

External endorsement responses to each item are:
1. b.
2. b.
3. a.
4. b.
5. a.
6. b.
7. a.
8. b.
9. a.
10. b.
11. b.
12. a.
13. a.
14. b.
15. a.
16. b.
17. b.
18. b.
19. a.
20. a.
21. b.
22. b.

23. a.
24. b.
25. a.

The DRIE is scored on the External direction by summing the number of external response options endorsed.

Total Score
Sum of external items endorsed across the entire scale.

Intrapersonal Factor
Sum of external endorsements on items #9, 11, 13, 14, 16, 17, 25

Interpersonal Factor
Sum of external endorsements on items #3, 4, 6, 7, 10, 22, 23

General Control Factor
Sum of external endorsements on items #5, 8, 20.

Interpretation

The DRIE is a 25-item self-report questionnaire presented in a forced choice format. It is adapted from the concept model and assessment method developed by Rotter to define an individual's beliefs about the extent to which the outcome of important life events are under personal control (internal locus of control) or under the influence of chance, fate, or powerful others (external locus of control). The DRIE assesses these beliefs specifically with respect to the individual's perceptions of control over alcohol, drinking behavior, and recovery. The scale is multidimensional, having empirically defined actors assessing perceived control over interpersonal, intrapersonal, and general factors associated with drinking. Alcohol-dependent individuals have been found to be more external in their drinking-related Locus of control than nondependent drinkers. An external locus of control is associated with more physical, social, and psychological impairment from drinking. The perception of control appears to become more internal over the course of alcohol treatment; individuals with more external perceptions are also more likely to drop out of treatment prematurely. Following treatment, alcoholics having an internal drinking related locus of control are less likely to relapse, drink less and have a shorter prolonged drinking episode if they do relapse, and have a better overall drinking-related outcome than alcoholics with an external DRIE score. The DRIE has been found to differentiate between alcohol dependent and nondependent individuals; to be related to drinking patterns and alcohol-related physical, social, and psychological impairment among alcohol-dependent individuals; and to be predictive of posttreatment drinking behavior.

Source: National Institutes for Health

The CAGE Questionnaire

The CAGE questionnaire is a simple but effective test designed to screen for alcohol abuse. It consists of four questions:

1. Have you ever felt the need to cut down on your drinking?
2. Do you feel annoyed by people complaining about your drinking?
3. Do you ever feel guilty about your drinking?
4. Do you ever drink an eye-opener in the morning to relieve the shakes?

Studies reveal that two "yes" answers to the CAGE questionnaire will correctly identify 75 percent of the alcoholics who respond to it and accurately eliminate 96 percent of nonalcoholics.

Alcohol Effects Questionnaire

Directions

We would like to find out what you personally experience after you have had a few alcoholic drinks. For the following possible experiences, if an item is always or sometimes true for you, circle true. If the item is rarely or never true for you, circle false. Please answer every question without skipping any.

True False 1. Drinking makes me feel flushed.

True False 2. Alcohol decreases muscular tension in my body.

True False 3. A few drinks make me feel less shy.

True False 4. Alcohol enables me to fall asleep more easily.

True False 5. I feel powerful when I drink, as if I can really influence others to do as I want.

True False 6. I'm more clumsy after a few drinks.

True False 7. I'm more romantic when I drink.

True False 8. Drinking makes the future seem brighter to me.

True False 9. If I have had a couple of drinks it is easier for me to tell someone off.

True False 10. I can't act as quickly when I've been drinking.

True False 11. Alcohol can act as an anesthetic for me, that is, it can deaden pain.

True False 12. I often feel sexier after I've had a few drinks.

True False 13. Drinking makes me feel good.

True False 14. Alcohol makes me careless about my actions.

True False 15. Some alcohol has a pleasant, cleansing, tingly taste to me.

True False 16. Drinking increases my aggressiveness.

True False 17. Alcohol seems like magic to me.

True False 18. Alcohol makes it hard for me to concentrate.

True False 19. I'm a better lover after a few drinks.

True False 20. When I'm drinking, it is easier to open up and express my feelings.

True False 21. Drinking adds a certain warmth to social occasions.

True False 22. If I'm feeling restricted in any way, a few drinks make me feel better.

True False 23. I can't think as quickly after I drink.

True False 24. Having a few drinks is a nice way for me to celebrate special occasions.

True False 25. Alcohol makes me worry less.

True False 26. Drinking makes me inefficient.

True False 27. Drinking is pleasurable because its enjoyable for me to join in with people who are enjoying themselves.

True False 28. After a few drinks, I am more sexually responsive.

True False 29. I feel more coordinated after I drink.

True False 30. I'm more likely to say embarrassing things after drinking.

True False 31. I enjoy having sex more if I've had some alcohol.

True False 32. I'm more likely to get into an argument if I've had some alcohol.

True False 33. Alcohol makes me less concerned about doing things well.

True False 34. Alcohol helps me sleep better.

True False 35. Drinking gives me more confidence in myself.

True False 36. Alcohol makes me more irresponsible.

True False 37. After a few drinks it is easier for me to pick a fight.

True False 38. A few drinks make it easier for me to talk to people.

True False 39. If I have a couple of drinks it is easier to express my feelings.

True False 40. Alcohol makes me more interesting.

Scoring

Each scale score is the sum of the following items that are marked "true." POS (items 8, 17, 22, 29, 40), SPP (items 13, 15, 21, 24, 27), SEX (items 7, 12, 19, 28, 31), AGG (items 1, 5, 9, 16, 32, 37), SOC (items 3, 20, 35, 38, 39), REL (items 2, 4, 11, 25, 34), IMP (6, 10, 18, 23, 26), and CU (14, 30, 33, 36).

The AEQ, a revision and extension of the Alcohol Expectancy Questionnaire by Brown et al. (1980), was developed as a brief method of assessing both the positive and negative effects people expect alcohol to have on themselves. It assesses undesirable effects of alcohol (impairment and irresponsibility) as well as reinforcing effects.

The AEQ was developed by taking the five items that loaded most highly on the six factors of the AEQ scale, adding two items assessing verbal aggression and deleting from the aggression scale one item that had loaded on two factors, adding five items assessing cognitive and physical impairment and four items assessing carelessness or lack of concern about consequences, then rewording all items to reflect personal beliefs. The scales are called: Global Positive (POS),
Social and Physical Pleasure (SPP), Sexual Enhancement (SEX), Power and Aggression (AGG), Social Expressiveness (SOC), Relaxation and Tension Reduction (REL), Cognitive and Physical Impairment (IMP), and Careless Unconcern (CU).

Among a sample of 85 male and 65 female college student drinkers of all levels of drinking (Rohsenow 1983), the mean percentage of items endorsed for each scale was POS 22 percent, SPP 82 percent, SEX 42 percent, AGG 51 percent, SOC 74 percent, REL 66 percent, IMP 72 percent, and CU 67 percent.

Among 87 alcoholics in treatment (Rohsenow et al. 1992), the mean percentage of items endorsed for each scale was POS 44 percent, SPP 76 percent, SEX 40 percent, AGG 59 percent, SOC 79 percent, REL 83 percent, IMP 69 percent, and CU 75 percent.

Rohsenow, D.J. Drinking habits and expectancies about alcohol's effects for self versus others. J Consult Clin Psychol 51:752-756, 1983.

Rohsenow, D.J.; Monti, P.M.; Abrams, D.B.; Rubonis, A.V.; Niaura, R.S.; Sirota, A.D.; and Colby, S.M. Cue elicited urge to drink and salivation in alcoholics: Relationship to individual differences. Adv Behav Res Ther 14:195-210,1992.

Source: National Institutes of Health, Alcohol Effects Questionnaire

Why Do You Smoke?

Directions

Indicate the degree to which each of the statements is true for you.

Never	Sometimes	Often	
			1. When I run out of cigarettes, it's almost unbearable until I get more.
			2. I am very aware of not smoking when I don't have a cigarette in my hand.
			3. When I haven't smoked for a while I get a gnawing hunger for a cigarette.
			4. I smoke to keep from slowing down
			5. I reach for a cigarette when I need a lift.
			6. When I'm tired, smoking perks me up.
			7. I smoke cigarettes automatically without being aware of it.
			8. I light up a cigarette without realizing I have one burning in an ashtray.
			9. I find a cigarette in my mouth and don't remember putting it there.
			10. Smoking cigarettes is pleasant and enjoyable.
			11. Smoking makes good times better.
			12. I want a cigarette most when I am comfortable and relaxed.
			13. I light up a cigarette when something makes me angry.
			14. Smoking relaxes me in a stressful situation.
			15. When I'm depressed I reach for a cigarette to feel better.
			16. I feel more comfortable with a cigarette in my hand.
			17. I enjoy getting a cigarette out of the pack and lighting up.
			18. I like to watch the smoke when I exhale.

Scoring

Smokers use tobacco to fill many different needs. Studies show that most people smoke for one or more of the following reasons:

1. Smoking gives me more energy.
2. I like to touch and handle cigarettes.
3. Smoking is a pleasure.
4. Smoking helps me relax when I'm tense or upset.
5. I crave cigarettes; smoking is an addiction.
6. Smoking is a habit.

If you answered "often" or "sometimes" to questions 4, 5, 6 then one of the reasons you smoke may be because smoking gives you more energy. Many people use tobacco like they use coffee: to help them wake up, get moving, keep going when they feel worn out. The nicotine in tobacco, like the caffeine in coffee, is a stimulant. But you can find other ways to get more energy.

If you answered "often" or "sometimes" to questions 16, 17, 18 then one of the reasons you smoke may be because you like to touch and handle cigarettes. This type of smoker gets physical pleasure from handling ciga- rettes and the rituals of smoking. It just "feels right" to have a cig- arette in his hand or mouth. In fact, many smokers say they've gone back to smoking because, "I had nothing to do with my hands."

If you answered "often" or "sometimes" to questions 10, 11, 12 then one of the reasons you smoke may be because smoking is a pleasure. Almost two out of three smokers say they just plain enjoy smoking. When you associate smoking with "the good times," it can strengthen your smoking habit. But it can be easier to quit when you focus on enjoying yourself without tobacco.

If you answered "often" or "sometimes" to questions 13, 14, 15 then one of the reasons you smoke may be because smoking helps you relax when I'm tense or upset. Lots of smokers use cigarettes to help them through bad times. If you've used cigarettes as a crutch, finding another.

If you answered "often" or "sometimes" to questions 1,2,3 then one of the reasons you smoke may be because you crave cigarettes and are addicted to smoking. Many smokers are addicted or "hooked" on the nicotine in tobacco. When addicted smokers quit, many go through a withdrawal period. They may have both physical symptoms (feeling tired and irritable; headaches; nervousness) and an emotional need for a cigarette.

If you answered "often" or "sometimes" to questions 7, 8, 9 then one of the reasons you smoke may be because smoking is a habit. If you are this kind of smoker, you are no longer getting much satisfaction from your cigarettes. Unlike people who smoke for pleasure, you might not miss it very much if you stopped. The key is breaking your smoking patterns.

Source: Developed from materials provided by the National Institutes of Health, National Cancer Institute, "Why Do You Smoke?"

Beliefs About Smoking

Directions

The sentences below are about how you might be affected by smoking. Put a check to show how much you agree or disagree with each sentence.

	Strongly Agree	Agree	Not Sure	Disagree	Strongly Disagree
1. 1 would have to smoke regularly for many years before smoking would affect my health.					
2. Smoking only a few cigarettes a day would hurt my health.					
3. People who smoke are more successful than those who don't smoke.					
4. Pipes and cigars are safe to smoke if I don't inhale.					
5. After quitting, ex-smokers will be as healthy as if they had never smoked.					
6. The health risks of smoking can be overcome through exercise.					
7. Social gatherings are better when people are smoking.					
8. Smoking cigarettes is a sign of being mature.					
9. Most people who smoke cigarettes can quit smoking whenever they want to.					

•

Scoring and Analysis

This affective measure assesses participants' belief in the value of not smoking.

Point values are assigned to responses according to the following scoring.

Item No.	Strongly Agree	Agree	Not Sure	Disagree	Strongly Disagree
1	1	2	3	4	5
2	5	4	3	2	1
3	1	2	3	4	5
4	1	2	3	4	5
5	1	2	3	4	5
6	1	2	3	4	5
7	1	2	3	4	5
8	1	2	3	4	5
9	1	2	3	4	5
10	1	2	3	4	5
11	1	2	3	4	5
12	1	2	3	4	5
13	5	4	3	2	1
14	5	4	3	2	1
15	1	2	3	4	5

This inventory can be scored by adding the point values of the responses from all participants and dividing this total by the number of responses.

Blank items should not be counted in the number of responses.

The maximum attainable score of 5 points indicates a strong belief in the negative effects of smoking. A minimum score of 1 suggests weak belief in the negative effects of smoking.

Check Your High Blood Pressure Prevention IQ

Directions

Circle either True or False.

True False 1. There is nothing you can do to prevent high blood pressure.

True False 2. If your mother or father has high blood pressure, you'll get it.

True False 3. Young adults don't get high blood pressure.

True False 4. High blood pressure has no symptoms.

True False 5. Stress causes high blood pressure.

True False 6. High blood pressure is not life-threatening.

True False 7. Blood pressure is high when it's at or over 140/90 mm Hg.

True False 8. If you're overweight, you are two to six times more likely to develop high blood pressure.

True False 9. You have to exercise vigorously every day to improve your blood pressure and heart health.

True False 10. Americans eat two to three times more salt and sodium than they need.

True False 11. Drinking alcohol lowers blood pressure.

True False 12. High blood pressure has no cure.

Scoring

1. FALSE
High blood pressure can be prevented with four steps: keep a healthy weight; become physically active; limit your salt and sodium use; and, if you drink alcoholic beverages, do so in moderation.

2. FALSE
You are more likely to get high blood pressure if it runs in your family, but that doesn't mean you must get it. Your chance of getting high blood pressure is also greater if you're older or an African American. But high blood pressure is NOT an inevitable part of aging and everyone can take steps to prevent the disease--the steps are given in answer 1.

3. FALSE
About 15 percent of those ages 18-39 are among the 50 million Americans with high blood pressure. Once you have high blood pressure you have it for the rest of your life. So start now to prevent it.

4. TRUE

High blood pressure, or "hypertension," usually has no symptoms. In fact it is often called the "silent killer." You can have high blood pressure and feel fine. That's why it's important to have your blood pressure checked--it's a simple test.

5. FALSE

Stress does make blood pressure go up but only temporarily. Ups and downs in blood pressure are normal. Run for a bus and your pressure rises; sleep and it drops. Blood pressure is the force of blood against the walls of arteries. Blood pressure becomes dangerous when it's always high. That harms your heart and blood vessels. So what does cause high blood pressure? In the vast majority of cases, a single cause is never found

6. FALSE

High blood pressure is the main cause of stroke and a factor in the development of heart disease and kidney failure.

7. TRUE

But even blood pressures slightly under 140/90 mm Hg can increase your risk of heart disease or stroke.

8. TRUE

As weight increases, so does blood pressure. It's important to stay at a healthy weight. If you need to reduce try to lose 1/2 to 1 pound a week. Choose foods low in fat (especially saturated fat) since fat is high in calories. Even if you're at a good weight, the healthiest way to eat is low fat, low cholesterol.

9. FALSE

Studies show that even a little physical activity helps prevent high blood pressure and strengthens your heart. Even among the overweight, those who are active have lower blood pressures than those who aren't. It's best to do some activity for 30 minutes most days. Walk, garden or bowl. If you don't have a 30-minute period, do something for 15 minutes twice a day. Every bit helps--so make activity part of your daily routine.

10. TRUE

Americans eat way too much salt and sodium. And some people, such as many African Americans, are especially sensitive to salt. Salt is made of sodium and chloride and it's mostly the sodium that affects blood pressure. Salt is only one form of sodium--there are others. So you need to watch your use of both salt and sodium. That includes what's added to foods at the table and in cooking and what's already in processed foods and snacks. Americans, especially people with high blood pressure, should eat no more than about 6 grams of salt a day, which equals about 2,400 milligrams of sodium.

11. FALSE

Drinking too much alcohol can raise blood pressure. If you drink have no more than two drinks a day. The "Dietary Guidelines" recommend that for overall health, women should limit their alcohol to no more than one drink a day. A drink would be 1.5 ounces of 80 proof whiskey, or 5 ounces of wine, or 12 ounces of beer.

12. TRUE
But high blood pressure can be treated and controlled. Treatment usually includes lifestyle changes--losing weight, if overweight; becoming physically active; limiting salt and sodium; and avoiding drinking excess alcohol--and, if needed, medication. But the best way to avoid the dangers of high blood pressure is to prevent the condition.

Source: U.S. Department of Health and Human Services, Public Health Service, National Institutes of Health, National Heart, Lung, and Blood Institute, HEALTHWise, October 1996

Check Your Healthy Heart I.Q.

Directions

Answer "true" or "false" to the following questions to test your knowledge of heart disease and its risk factors.

True False 1. The risk factors for heart disease that you can do something about are: high blood pressure, high blood cholesterol, smoking, obesity, and physical inactivity.

True False 2. A stroke is often the first symptom of high blood pressure, and a heart attack is often the first symptom of high blood cholesterol.

True False 3. A blood pressure greater than or equal to 140/90 mm Hg is generally considered to be high.

True False 4. High blood pressure affects the same number of blacks as it does whites.

True False 5. The best ways to treat and control high blood pressure are to control your weight, exercise, eat less salt (sodium), restrict your intake of alcohol, and take your high blood pressure medicine, if prescribed by your doctor.

True False 6. A blood cholesterol of 240 mg/dL is desirable for adults.

True False 7. The most effective dietary way to lower the level of your blood cholesterol is to eat foods low in cholesterol.

True False 8. Lowering blood cholesterol levels can help people who have already had a heart attack.

True False 9. Only children from families at high risk of heart disease need to have their blood cholesterol levels checked.

True False 10. Smoking is a major risk factor for four of the five leading causes of death including heart attack, stroke, cancer, and lung diseases such as emphysema and bronchitis.

True False 11. If you have had a heart attack, quitting smoking can help reduce your chances of having a second attack.

True False 12. Someone who has smoked for 30 to 40 years probably will not be able to quit smoking.

True False 13. The best way to lose weight is to increase physical activity and eat fewer calories.

True False 14. Heart disease is the leading killer of men and women in the United States.

Scoring

Compare your responses with the correct quiz answers and explanations that follow:

1. TRUE

High blood pressure, smoking, and high blood cholesterol are the three most important risk factors for heart disease. On the average, each one doubles your chance of developing heart disease. So, a person who has all three of the risk factors is 8 times more likely to develop heart disease than someone who has none. Obesity increases the likelihood of developing high blood cholesterol and high blood pressure, which increase your risk of heart disease. Physical inactivity increases your risk for heart attack. Regular exercise and good nutrition are essential to reducing high blood pressure, high blood cholesterol, and overweight. People who exercise are also more likely to cut down or stop smoking.

2. TRUE

A person with high blood pressure or high blood cholesterol may feel fine and look great; there are often no signs that anything is wrong until a stroke or heart attack occurs. To find out if you have high blood pressure or high blood cholesterol, you should be tested by a doctor, nurse, or other health professional.

3. TRUE

A blood pressure of 140/90 mm Hg or greater is generally classified as high blood pressure. However, blood pressures that fall below 140/90 mmHg can sometimes be a problem. If the diastolic pressure, the second or lower number, is between 85-89, a person is at an increased risk for heart disease or stroke and should have his/her bloodpressure checked at least once a year by a health professional. The higher your blood pressure, the greater your risk of developing heart disease or stroke. Controlling high blood pressure reduces your risk.

4. FALSE

High blood pressure is more common in blacks than whites. It affects 29 out of every 100 black adults compared to 26 out of every 100 white adults. Also, with aging, high blood pressure is generally more severe among blacks then among whites, and therefore causes more strokes, heart disease, and kidney failure.

5. TRUE

Recent studies show that lifestyle changes can help keep blood pressure levels normal even into advanced age and are important in treating and preventing high blood pressure. Limit high-salt foods which include many snack foods, such as potato chips, salted pretzels, and salted crackers; processed foods, such as canned soups; and condiments, such as ketchup and soy sauce. Also, it is extremely important to take blood pressure medication, if prescribed by your doctor, to make sure your blood pressure stays under control.

6. FALSE

A total blood cholesterol of under 200 mg/dL is desirable and usually puts you at a lower risk for heart disease. A blood cholesterol level of 240 mg/dL or above is high and increases your risk of heart disease. If your cholesterol level is high, your doctor will want to check your levels of LDL-cholesterol ("bad" cholesterol) and HDL- cholesterol ("good" cholesterol). A HIGH level of LDL-cholesterol increases your risk for heart disease, as does a LOW level of HDL-cholesterol. A cholesterol level of 200-239 mg/dL is considered borderline-high and usually increases your risk for heart disease. If your cholesterol is borderline-high, you should speak to your doctor to see if additional cholesterol tests are needed. All adults 20 years of age or older should have their blood cholesterol level checked at least once every 5 years.

7. FALSE

Reducing the amount of cholesterol in your diet is important; however, eating foods low in saturated fat is the most effective dietary way to lower blood cholesterol levels, along with eating less total fat and cholesterol. Choose low-saturated fat foods, such as grains, fruits, and vegetables; low-fat or skim milk and milk products; lean cuts of meat; fish; and chicken. Trim fat from meat before cooking; bake or broil meat rather than fry; use less fat and oil; and take the skin off chicken and turkey. Reducing overweight will also help lower your level of LDL- cholesterol as well as increase your level of HDL- cholesterol.

8. TRUE

People who have had one heart attack are at much higher risk for a second attack. Reducing blood cholesterol levels can greatly slow down (and, in some people, even reverse) the buildup of cholesterol and fat in the walls of the arteries and significantly reduce the chances of a second heart attack.

9. TRUE

Children from "high risk" families, in which a parent has high blood cholesterol (240 mg/dL or above) or in which a parent or grandparent has had heart disease at an early age (at 55 years of age or younger), should have their cholesterol levels tested. If a child from such a family has a cholesterol level that is high, it should be lowered under medical supervision, primarily with diet, to reduce the risk of developing heart disease as an adult. For most children, who are not from high-risk families, the best way to reduce the risk of adult heart disease is to follow a low-saturated fat, low cholesterol eating pattern. All children over the age of 2 years and all adults should adopt a heart-healthy eating pattern as a principal way of reducing coronary heart disease.

10. TRUE

Heavy smokers are 2 to 4 times more likely to have a heart attack than nonsmokers, and the heart attack death rate among all smokers is 70 percent greater than that of nonsmokers. Older male smokers are also nearly twice as likely to die from stroke than older men who do not smoke, and these odds are nearly as high for older female smokers. Further, the risk of dying from lung cancer is 22 times higher for male smokers than male nonsmokers and 12 times higher for female smokers than female nonsmokers. Finally, 80 percent of all deaths from emphysema and bronchitis are directly due to smoking.

11. TRUE

One year after quitting, ex-smokers cut their extra risk for heart attack by about half or more, and eventually the risk will return to normal in healthy ex-smokers. Even if you have already had a heart attack, you can reduce your chances of a second attack if you quit smoking. Ex-smokers can also reduce their risk of smoke and cancer, improve blood flow and lung function, and help stop diseases like emphysema and bronchitis from getting worse.

12. FALSE
Older smokers are more likely to succeed at quitting smoking than younger smokers. Quitting helps relieve smoking-related symptoms like shortness of breath, coughing, and chest pain. Many quit to avoid further health problems and take control of their lives.

13. TRUE
Weight control is a question of balance. You get calories from the foods you eat. You burn off calories by exercising. Cutting down on calories, especially calories from fat, is key to losing weight. Combining this with a regular physical activity, like walking, cycling, jogging, or swimming, not only can help in losing weight but also in maintaining weight loss. A steady weight loss of 1/2 to 1 pounds a week is safe for most adults, and the weight is more likely to stay off over the long run. Losing weight, if you are overweight, may also reduce your blood pressure, lower your LDL-cholesterol, and raise your HDL- cholesterol. Being physically active and eating fewer calories will also help you control your weight if you quit smoking.

14. TRUE
Coronary heart disease is the #1 killer in the United States. Approximately 489,000 Americans died of coronary heart disease in 1990, and approximately half of the deaths were women.

Source: U.S. Department of Health and Human Services, Public Health Service, NATIONAL INSTITUTES OF HEALTH
Revised October 1992, Updated August 1996

Your Risks of STDs

Name: ______________________________ Date: ____________

Directions: For each category below, circle the *one* answer that best describes you, your attitudes, and/or your behavior.

AGE

Age	*Points if Male*	*Points if Female*
0-10	1	1
11-14	2	3
15-19	4	6
20-30	5	4
31-35	3	3
36+	2	2

SEXUAL PREFERENCE

Preference	*Points*
Celibate	0
Heterosexual	3
Bisexual	6
Gay male, multiple partners	8
Gay female	1
Gay male, monogamous	5

NUMBER OF PARTNERS

Number	*Points*
Never engage in sex	0
One sex partner only	1
More than one sex partner, but never more than one relationship at a time	2
2-5 sex partners	4
5-10 sex partners	6
10+ sex partners	8

SEXUAL ATTITUDES

Attitude	*Points*
Will not engage in non-marital sex	0
Monogamous relationship only	1
Sex OK if relationship is long-term	1
An occasional fling OK	4
Sex OK with multiple or casual partners	8
Believe in *complete* sexual freedom	8

ATTITUDES TOWARD CONTRACEPTION

Attitude	*Points*
Not now sexually active	0
Would use condom to prevent pregnancy	1
Would use condom with all but steady partner	2
Would not use condom ever	6
Self or partner would use the pill	5
Would use other contraceptive measures	4
Sexually active and use nothing, but don't worry about STDs or pregnancy	8

ATTITUDES TOWARD STDs

Attitude	*Points*
Not now sexually active, so no need to worry	1
Would definitely tell my partner(s) if I had an STD	2
Would see a doctor at first sign of symptoms	2
Would wait to see if symptoms go away	6
Am sexually active, but low risk because all partners are clean	6
STDs no sweat because I know I'll never have it.	5

Scoring: Total the points circled.

Interpretation:

5-10	Well below average
11-15	Below average
16-20	Average
21-24	Moderate risk
25+	High risk

Check Your Asthma I.Q.

Directions

The following true-or-false statements test what you know about asthma.

True False 1. Asthma is a common disease among children and adults in the United States.

True False 2. Asthma is an emotional or psychological illness.

True False 3. The way that parents raise their children can cause asthma.

True False 4. Asthma episodes may cause breathing problems, but these episodes are not really harmful or dangerous.

True False 5. Asthma episodes usually occur suddenly without warning.

True False 6. Many different things can bring on an asthma episode.

True False 7. Asthma cannot be cured, but it can be controlled.

True False 8. There are different types of medicine to control asthma.

True False 9. People with asthma have no way to monitor how well their lungs are functioning.

True False 10. Both children and adults can have asthma.

True False 11. Tobacco smoke can make an asthma episode worse.

True False 12. People with asthma should not exercise.

Scoring

11-12 correct = Congratulations! You know a lot about asthma. Share this information with your family and friends.

10-11 correct = Very good.

Fewer than 10 correct = Go over the answers and try to learn more about asthma.

Answers to the Asthma "I.Q." Quiz

1. TRUE.
Asthma is a common disease among children and adults in the United States, and it is increasing. About 10 million people have asthma, of whom 3 million are under 18 years of age.

2. FALSE.
Asthma is not an emotional or psychological disease, although strong emotions can sometimes make asthma worse. People with asthma have sensitive lungs that react to certain things, causing the airways to tighten, swell, and fill with mucus. The person then has trouble breathing and may cough and wheeze.

3. FALSE.
The way parents raise their children does not cause asthma. It is not caused by a poor parent-child relationship or by being overprotective.

4. FALSE.
Asthma episodes can be very harmful. People can get very sick and need hospitalization. Some people have died from asthma episodes. Frequent asthma episodes, even if they are mild, may cause people to stop being active and living normal lives.

5. FALSE.
Sometimes an asthma episode may come on quite quickly. However, before a person has any wheezing or shortness of breath there are usually symptoms such as a cough, a scratchy throat, or tightness in the chest. Most patients learn to recognize these early symptoms and can take medicine to prevent a serious episode.

6. TRUE.
For most people with asthma, an episode can start from many different "triggers." Some of these things are pollen from trees or grasses; molds or house dust; weather changes; strong odors; cigarette smoke; and certain foods. Other triggers include being upset; laughing or crying hard; having a cold or the flu; or being near furry or feathered animals. Each person with asthma has an individual set of asthma "triggers."

7. TRUE.
There is no cure yet for asthma. However, asthma patients can control it to a large degree by:
Getting advice from a doctor who treats asthma patients
Learning to notice early signs of an asthma episode and to start treatment.
Avoiding things that cause asthma episodes.
Taking medicine just as the doctor says.
Knowing when to get medical help with a severe episode.

8. TRUE.
Several types of medicines are available to control asthma. Some people with mild asthma need to take medication only when they have symptoms. But most people need to take medicine every day to prevent symptoms and also to take medicine when symptoms do occur. A doctor needs to decide the best type of medicine for each patient and how often it should be taken. Asthma patients and their doctors need to work together to manage the disease.

9. FALSE.
People with asthma can monitor how well their lungs are functioning with a peak flow meter. This small device can be used at home, work, or school. The peak flow meter may show that the asthma is getting worse before the usual symptoms appear.

10. TRUE.
Both children and adults can have asthma. Sometimes, but not always, symptoms will go away as children get older. However, many children continue to have asthma symptoms throughout adulthood. In some cases, symptoms of asthma are not recognized until a person is an adult.

11. TRUE.
Smoke from cigarettes, cigars and pipes can bring on an asthma attack. Indoor smoky air from fireplaces and outdoor smog can make asthma worse. Some can also "set off" other triggers. Smokers should be asked not to smoke near someone with asthma. Moving to another room may help, but smoke travels room to room. No smoking is best for everyone!

12. FALSE.
Exercise is good for most people--with or without asthma. When asthma is under good control, people with asthma are able to play most sports. For people whose asthma is brought on by exercise, medicines can be taken before exercising to help avoid an episode. A number of Olympic medalists have asthma.

Source: CHECK YOUR ASTHMA "I.Q.", National Asthma Education Program, National Heart, Lung, and Blood Institute, National Institutes of Health, Reprinted October 1992

Check Your Blood I.Q.

Directions

The following "true-or-false" statements test what you know about blood.

True False 1. Just 1 pint of your blood can help save the lives of several people.

True False 2. Giving blood is a simple process.

True False 3. Artificial or animal blood can now be used in place of human blood.

True False 4. Filling out the blood donor forms honestly and completely is a very important part of the process of giving blood.

True False 5. You cannot get AIDS or any other disease by donating blood.

True False 6. Most donors are paid money for their blood.

True False 7. It is best to wait until a friend needs blood before donating.

True False 8. Some people can donate blood for their own use.

True False 9. The Nation's blood supply is safer than ever before.

True False 10. Giving blood more than once a year will make you weak.

True False 11. The chance of getting AIDS from blood transfusions is very low.

Scoring

Answers to the Blood "I.Q." Quiz

1. TRUE.
The pint of blood you donate is usually split into several parts to meet the needs of different patients. For example, your platelets may give a child with leukemia a chance to live, while your red cells may help an accident victim get well. Your single donation can help several patients.

2. TRUE.
Giving blood is simple and easy. You can expect to follow four steps: registration, medical history, donation, and snacks. The actual blood donation takes less than 10 minutes and is painless except for a little hurt at the very start. The entire process, from when you sign in to the time you leave, takes about 45 minutes.

3. FALSE.
There is no substitute for human blood. Human blood can not be manufactured; animal blood can not replace it. People are the only source of blood. Much of today's medical care depends on a steady supply of blood provided by healthy donors. The gift of blood is the gift of life.

4. TRUE.
It is very important to complete the blood donor forms honestly. People who should not donate need to identified before the blood is taken. All information given by the donor is treated confidentially.

5. TRUE.
There is no risk of getting AIDS or any other disease from giving blood. A brand new needle is used for each blood donation. Once it is used, the needle is destroyed.

6. FALSE.
Volunteers now provide virtually all of the Nation's blood supply. This represents a huge increase in volunteer donations over the past 10 years. People donate blood out of a sense of duty and community spirit, not to make money.

7. FALSE.
Many tests must be done before blood can be used. For emergencies, there is no time to collect, test, and process the blood from friends. Having enough blood on hand when we need it is possible only if healthy volunteers donate blood regularly.

8. TRUE.
For planned surgery, it is often possible to donate your own blood ahead of time so that it will be available for your operation if needed. It also may be possible for a surgeon to collect blood from a wound during an operation and return it to the patient. Both are forms of autologous transfusion. It is the safest kind of transfusion, but most patients needed blood cannot provide their own. Therefore, there remains a great need for healthy people to donate blood for others. For information on whether you can donate blood for your own use, ask your doctor.

9. TRUE.
The risk of getting unsafe blood from a transfusion has been greatly reduced. Blood collection centers help to protect the blood supply by constantly improving safety measures. For example, they: inform donors about high-risk behaviors and conditions that are not safe for blood donation; allow anyone to indicate confidentially that their blood should not be used for the general blood supply; take a medical history to check that donors are healthy; collect blood using sterile methods under medical supervision; and test blood for certain diseases.

10. FALSE.
Giving blood will not decrease your strength. Your body won't miss the 1 pint of blood you donate. Healthy donors can give blood as often as every 8 weeks. If all blood donors gave at least twice a year, it would greatly strengthen the Nation's blood supply.

11. TRUE.
The risk of getting AIDS from blood transfusions is extremely low. Necessary blood transfusions can save lives; therefore, the benefits are much greater than the risks. Ask your doctor for more information about blood transfusions.

Source: National Blood Resources Education Program, National Heart, Lung, and Blood Institute, NATIONAL INSTITUTES OF HEALTH, September 1988

Chronic Fatigue Syndrome Symptoms Checklist

Indicate if any of the following symptoms began at, or after, the onset of illness and have persisted or recurred during a 6-month period:

____ 1. mild fever (99.5°_101.5° F) and/or chills
____ 2. sore throat
____ 3. painful lymph nodes
____ 4. muscular discomfort
____ 5. prolonged (24 hours) generalized fatigue after exercise that was easily tolerated before illness
____ 6. generalized headaches (different from those you had before illness)
____ 7. migratory arthralgia (pain) without joint swelling or redness
____ 8. psychological complaints (e.g., forgetfulness, excessive irritability, confusion, depression)
____ 9. sleep disturbance
____ 10. sudden onset of symptoms (considered to be of equal importance as the symptoms)
____ 11. unexplained generalized muscle weakness

Scoring

Add the total number of symptoms you indicated. When all other conditions that might have caused the fatigue are ruled-out, a diagnosis may be made if you have experienced at least 6 of these 11 symptoms that began at, or after, the onset of illness and have persisted or recurred during a 6-month period.

The etiologic agent that causes Chronic Fatigue Syndrome (CFS) is unknown. No specific diagnostic tests have been developed for identifying CFS. Because incapacitating fatigue can be associated with a wide range of well-defined illnesses, a diagnosis of CFS is made by a process of elimination. In the United States, the majority of diagnosed cases of CFS occur in white women, 25_45 years of age.

Source: Adapted from Facts about Chronic Fatigue Syndrome, Centers for Disease Control and Prevention, February1997

How Accurate Are Your Perceptions of Aging?

Name: ______________________________ Date: __________

Directions: Indicate whether each of the following questions is true or false about the aged (defined as those over 65).

___ 1. The majority of the aged are senile.

___ 2. The majority of the aged only seldom become irritated or angry.

___ 3. Most of the aged have no interest in, or capacity for, sexual relations.

___ 4. Lung capacity tends to decline in old age.

___ 5. Most of the aged feel miserable all the time.

___ 6. Physical strength tends to decline in old age.

___ 7. Most of the aged live in extended care institutions (nursing homes, mental hospitals, etc.).

___ 8. Aged drivers have fewer accidents per person than drivers under age 65.

___ 9. Most older workers cannot work as effectively as younger workers.

___ 10. The vast majority of the aged are healthy enough to carry out their normal activities.

___ 11. Most of the aged are set in their ways and cannot change.

___ 12. Old people usually take longer to learn something new.

___ 13. It is almost impossible for the aged to learn new things.

___ 14. The reaction of most older people tends to be slower than the reaction of most younger people.

___ 15. In general, most of the aged are pretty much alike.

___ 16. The majority of the aged are seldom bored.

___ 17. The majority of the aged are socially isolated and lonely.

___ 18. Older workers have fewer accidents than younger workers.

___ 19. The health and socioeconomic status of older people (compared to younger people) in the year 2000 will probably be about the same as that of today's older people.

___ 20. Most medical practitioners tend to give low priority to the aged.

___ 21. The majority of the aged have incomes below the poverty level (as defined by the federal government).

___ 22. The majority of the aged are working or would like to have some kind of work to do (including housework and volunteer work).

___ 23. Older people tend to become more religious as they age.

Scoring: Compare your responses with the following answer key and add up the number of wrong answers you scored.

Answer key: All odd-numbered statements are false; all even-numbered statements are true.

Interpretation: The more wrong answers you got, the more likely it is that you have a negative view of aging and the aged. Unless you plan to die young, reconsider aging in terms of what senior citizens *can* do.

Source: Dr. Erdman Palmore, Duke University Center for the Study of Aging and Human Development, Durham, NC. Initially published in The Gerontologist, Vol. 20, No. 6, 1980.

I'd Pick More Daisies

Name: ____ Date: ____________

If I had my life to live over,
I'd try to make more mistakes next time.
I would relax. I would limber up.
I would be sillier than I have been on this trip.
I would be crazier, I would be less hygienic.
I know of very few things I would take seriously.
I would take more chances. I would take more trips.
I would climb more mountains, swim more rivers, and watch more sunsets.
I would burn more gasoline.
I would eat more ice cream, less beans.
I would have more actual troubles and fewer imaginary ones.
You see, I am one of those sensible people who lives sensibly and sanely,
hour after hour, day after day.
Oh, I've had my moments.
And, if I had it to do over again, I'd have more of them.
In fact, I'd try to have nothing else.
Just moments, one after another,
Instead of living so many years ahead each day.
I have been one of those people who never go anywhere without a
thermometer, a hot water bottle, a gargle, a raincoat, a parachute.
If I had it to do over again I would go places and do things, and travel
lighter than I have.
If I had my life to live over, I would start barefooted earlier in the
spring, and stay that way later in the fall,
I would play hooky more.
I wouldn't make such good grades except by accident.
I would ride more merry-go-rounds.
I'd pick more daisies.

Anonymous

React to this poem: ____

____

____

____

____

____

____

____

____

____

____

Ten Ways To Recognize Hearing Loss

Directions

The following questions will help you determine if you need to have your hearing evaluated by a medical professional:

Yes No Do you have a problem hearing over the telephone?

Yes No Do you have trouble following the conversation when two or more people are talking at the same time?

Yes No Do people complain that you turn the TV volume up too high?

Yes No Do you have to strain to understand conversation?

Yes No Do you have trouble hearing in a noisy background?

Yes No Do you find yourself asking people to repeat themselves?

Yes No Do many people you talk to seem to mumble (or not speak clearly)?

Yes No Do you misunderstand what others are saying and respond inappropriately?

Yes No Do you have trouble understanding the speech of women and children?

Yes No Do people get annoyed because you misunderstand what they say?

Scoring

If you answered "yes" to three or more of these questions, you may want to see an otolaryngologist (an ear, nose, and throat specialist) or an audiologist for a hearing evaluation.

The material on this page is for general information only and is not intended for diagnostic or treatment purposes. A doctor or other health care professional must be consulted for diagnostic information and advice regarding treatment.

Source: National Institute on Deafness and Other Communication Disorders, National Institutes of Health, 31 Center Drive, MSC 2320, Bethesda, MD USA 20892-2320

Take this Eye-Q Test

Directions

Fifty million Americans are at risk for vision loss from glaucoma, a leading cause of blindness in the United States. Are you one of them? If you are, do you know how to reduce your risk of blindness? To determine how high your Eye-Q is, answer the following questions about glaucoma.

True	False	Not Sure	1. Glaucoma is more common in Blacks than in Whites.
True	False	Not Sure	2. Glaucoma tends to run in families.
True	False	Not Sure	3. A person can have glaucoma and not know it.
True	False	Not Sure	4. People over age 60 are more likely to get glaucoma.
True	False	Not Sure	5. Eye pain is often a symptom of glaucoma.
True	False	Not Sure	6. Glaucoma can be controlled.
True	False	Not Sure	7. Glaucoma is caused by increased eye pressure.
True	False	Not Sure	8. Vision lost from glaucoma can be restored.
True	False	Not Sure	9. A complete glaucoma exam consists only of measuring eye pressure.
True	False	Not Sure	10. People at risk for glaucoma should have an eye examination through dilated pupils.

Scoring

If you got 9 or 10 right, congratulations. You know a lot about glaucoma. If you missed some, review the answers so you can share your knowledge with your family and friends.

Answers

1. True.
In a study funded by the National Eye Institute, researchers at The Johns Hopkins University reported that glaucoma is three to four times more likely to occur in Blacks than in Whites. In addition, glaucoma is six times more likely to cause blindness in Blacks than in Whites.

2. True.
Although glaucoma tends to run in families, a hereditary basis has not been established. If someone in your immediate family has glaucoma, you should have your eyes examined through dilated pupils at least every two years.

3. True.
The early stages of open-angle glaucoma, the most common form, usually have no warning signs. However, as the disease progresses, a person with glaucoma may notice his or her side vision gradually failing.

4. True.
Everyone over age 60 has an increased risk for glaucoma. Other groups at increased risk include Blacks over age 40 and people with a family history of the disease.

5. False.
People with glaucoma usually do not experience pain from the disease.

6. True.
Although glaucoma cannot be cured, it usually can be controlled by eyedrops or pills, conventional surgery, or laser surgery. Sometimes eye care professionals will recommend a combination of surgery and medication.

7. True.
In glaucoma, for reasons still not completely understood, fluid drains too slowly out of the eye. As the fluid builds up, the pressure inside the eye rises. Unless this pressure is controlled, it may cause damage to the optic nerve and other parts of the eye and loss of vision.

8. False.
Vision loss from glaucoma is permanent. However, with early detection and treatment, the progression of visual loss can be slowed, or halted, and the risk of blindness reduced.

9. False.
A measurement of eye pressure by tonometry, though an important part of a comprehensive eye exam, is by itself not sufficient for the detection of glaucoma. Glaucoma is detected most often during an eye examination through dilated pupils. This means drops are put into the eyes during the exam to enlarge the pupils, which allows the eye care professional to see more of the inside of the eye to check for signs of glaucoma. When indicated, a visual field test should also be performed.

10. True.
An eye examination through dilated pupils is the best way to diagnose glaucoma.
Individuals at increased risk for the disease should have their eyes examined through dilated pupils at least every two years by an eye care professional.

Source: National Eye Health Education Program, National Eye Institute, National Institutes of Health, Revised 8–99

Death and Life's Human Relationships

Name: ______________________________________ Date: __________

Purpose: To make better use of human relationships by considering them finite.

Directions:

1. List fifteen people with whom you like to spend time.
2. Place an O next to anyone older than 50.
3. Place a Y next to anyone younger than 10.
4. Place a D next to the five people most likely to die first.
5. Place a T next to the five people you would most trust in a life-and-death situation.
6. Think of your three most valuable possessions. Place a G next to the three people to whom you would give one of these possessions if you were to die today.
7. If you were told you were dying and could only say goodbye to five of the people on your list, who would they be? Place an M next to these people.

	Name						
1.							
2.							
3.							
4.							
5.							
6.							
7.							
8.							
9.							
10.							
11.							
12.							
13.							
14.							
15.							

Results: Silently contemplate your responses to each of these questions:

1. Can you think of other people you would like to add to your list? Who are they? Why did you not include them originally?
2. Do you enjoy spending time with younger people, people your own age, or older people? Why?

3. Relative to the five people you identified as most likely to die first:
   a) Are they the oldest on your list?
   b) Do you now want to spend more time with them?
   c) What do you want to do with them before they die?
   d) Do you think they would guess that you would include them on such a list? Should you tell them you did?
4. If you were dying in a hospital, would you want any of the five people you designated as the ones you most trust to decide when to "pull the plug"? Or is there someone else to whom you would rather assign that responsibility?
5. How would you feel giving one of your most valued possessions to the people you designated with a G *now* rather than when you are dying? Would the meaning behind the gift be more valuable to you than the possession itself?

The class should then discuss what they have learned from this activity and how their behavior will be changed (if at all).

Source: Adapted from Jerrold S. Greenberg, Student-Centered Health Instruction: A Humanistic Approach. Reading, MA: Addison-Wesley, 1978. 246-47.

Environmental Quiz

Directions

Answer each question from the list of choices.

1. Which pollutants come from mobile sources?
   A. Hydrocarbons (Paraffins, Olefins, Naphthenes, Aromatics)
   B. Nitrogen Oxides (NO, NOx, NO_2)
   C. Carbon Dioxide (CO_2)
   D. Carbon Monoxide (CO)
   E. Particulates (any material collected on a filtering medium after exhaust dilution)
   F. Air Toxics
   G. None of the Above
   H. All of the Above

2. The combination of nitrogen oxides and hydrocarbons in the presence of sunlight causes:
   A. global Warming.
   B. smog (ozone).
   C. stratospheric Ozone Depletion.
   D. acid Rain.

3. Ozone is beneficial to our environment at high altitudes, yet harmful at low altitudes?
   A. TRUE
   B. FALSE

4. During the last 20 years, average ambient air levels of ozone, carbon monoxide, and lead have:
   A. gone up 10 percent.
   B. gone up 50 percent.
   C. not changed.
   D. gone down.

5. Which mobile source pollutant can not be controlled by emission control technology?
   A. Ozone forming hydrocarbons (C_nH_{2n+2})
   B. Carbon Monoxide (CO)
   C. Carbon Dioxide (CO_2)
   D. Air Toxics
   E. Particulate Matter (solid emissions)

6. Tailpipe exhaust is not always the greatest source of vehicle emissions?
   A. TRUE
   B. FALSE

7. Which of these vehicle fuels causes the least pollution?
   A. Electricity
   B. Reformulated Gasoline
   C. Natural Gas
   D. Alcohol
   E. Hydrogen
   F. Beer

8. What region of the US has experienced the worst effects from acid rain?
   A. North West
   B. North East
   C. South West
   D. South East

9. Which of the following is the biggest polluter of our air?
   A. City Buses
   B. Passenger Cars and Light Trucks
   C. Over-the-Road Trucks
   D. Power Plants

10. Estuaries suffer some of the worst effects of water and air pollution. Which of the following best describes an Estuary?
    A. The area where fresh water and salt water meet.
    B. A large inland body of water.
    C. An ancient river bed.
    D. None of the above

11. The largest contributor of NEW toxic pollution to the upper Great Lakes is:
    A. air Pollutants.
    B. sewage Treatment Plants
    C. factories

12. Which of the following is the source of Radon in homes?
    A. Ultraviolet Radiation
    B. Defective Heating Systems
    C. Uranium in Rock Formations
    D. None of the above

13. Where is there most potential for future gains in reducing motor vehicle emissions?
    A. Better control of emissions from vehicles in actual use
    B. Use of clean transportation alternatives such as mass transit
    C. Use of cleaner fuels
    D. All of the above

Scoring

1. Answer H. All of the Above

Right! All of these mobile source emissions can lead to air pollution. However, the near-complete switch to unleaded gasoline in this country has nearly eliminated lead as an ambient air quality problem in the United States.

2. Answer: B. Smog!

Ground-level ozone, otherwise known as urban smog. This is one of the most difficult air pollution problems to correct.

3. Answer: A. This statement is True!

At high altitudes, ozone acts as a shield against harmful ultraviolet radiation from the sun. At ground level, ozone can cause respiratory ailments in people and adverse effects on plant life.

4. Answer: D. They've Gone Down!

Levels of lead have gone down more than 90%! The phase-down of lead from gasoline has resulted in near elimination of lead emissions. Improvements in vehicle and emission control technology have also greatly reduced emissions of carbon monoxide, as well as ozone forming nitrogen oxides and hydrocarbons.

5. Answer: C. Carbon Dioxide - CO2!

CO2 is the ultimate result of perfect combustion of any carbon-based fuel. The only ways to reduce CO2 emissions are... to make vehicles more fuel efficient and/or drive less, to use a non-carbon fuel such as Hydrogen, to use a "green" fuel such as ethanol which is produced from crops that absorb CO2 as they grow. The Greenhouse Effect is caused by Carbon Dioxide and other gases absorbing infrared radiation in the atmosphere and warming the earth.

6. Answer: A. TRUE!

Vapors from evaporating gasoline, or "evaporative emissions", can account for two-thirds of the hydrocarbon emissions from gasoline-fueled vehicles on hot summer days. Evaporative emissions occur during vehicle refueling, vehicle operation, and even when the vehicle is parked.

7. Answer: E. Hydrogen!

While all of these fuels are cleaner than today's gasolines, hydrogen is the only one with the potential to be pollution-free, emitting only water vapor. However, hydrogen technology is decades away from being commercially viable. Battery-powered electric vehicles have the potential to emit zero pollution, but the power plants that generate electricity to charge the batteries do pollute.

8. Answer: B. North East

The most serious effects of acid rain have thus far been observed in the Northeast.

9. Answer: B. Passenger Cars and Light Trucks

There are over 200 million passenger cars and light trucks on American roads!
These vehicles drive almost 2 trillion miles every year.
Motor vehicles account for about 50% of air pollution nationwide.
The vehicle contribution to pollution is usually even higher in polluted cities.

10. Answer: A. Yes! Estuaries are the areas where fresh and salt water meet.

Some well-known examples of estuaries are: Chesapeake Bay, Puget Sound, San Francisco Bay.

11. Answer: A. The correct answer is AIR POLLUTANTS!

Research indicates that atmospheric sources are the single largest contributor of new toxic pollution to the upper Great Lakes, and a significant source, perhaps 20% in the lower Great Lakes. Acid rain threatens the Common Loon, duck populations, and other species of fish-eating birds. Research has implicated airborne sulfates in at least 50,000 premature deaths each year - as many lives as are lost in automobile accidents.

12. Answer: C. Uranium in Rock Formations

Radon is formed by the radioactive decay of uranium in naturally occurring rock formations, which could be located under your home.

13. Answer: D. All of the above!

You can do your part by making sure your vehicle is maintained properly, by choosing the most fuel efficient model that meets your needs, and using more efficient alternative transportation whenever possible, such as bike, carpool or mass transit.

Source: The Environmental Quiz, The U.S. Environmental Protection Agency, Office of Mobile Sources, National Vehicle and Fuel Emissions Laboratory, 18 May 1998.

Checklist for the Prevention of Carbon Monoxide (CO) Poisoning

Directions

The following questions relating to various areas in your environment will help you in dealing properly with the unseen, deadly hazard of carbon monoxide. The questions have been divided into sections that may directly apply to your particular situation. Most questions will apply equally to homeowners, campers, and to those who rent. Renters, however, should refer to the management any questions regarding maintenance. Draw a circle around your answer.

Yes No 1. Have you had the fireplace draft and the drafts of other fuel-burning appliances checked by an expert within the past year?

Yes No 2. Have all gas appliances been checked annually for proper operation?

Yes No 3. Are all Combustion appliances properly vented?

Yes No 4. Has your chimney vent been checked for defects within the past year?

Yes No 5. Have you patched any vent pipe with tape, gum, or other substances?

Yes No 6. Are all horizontal vent pipes to fuel appliances perfectly level?

Yes No 7. Do you use your gas range or oven for heating?

Yes No 8. Does the cooling unit of your gas refrigerator give off an odor?

Yes No 9. Have you ever used a charcoal grill, such as a barbecue grill for cooking within your home, cabin or camper other than in a vented fireplace?

Yes No 10. Have you ever brought burning charcoal into your home, cabin or camper for heating purposes?

Yes No 11. Do you consider portable flameless chemical heaters (catalytic) safe for use in your cabin, camper or home?

Yes No 12. Have you ever used a portable gas camp stove in your home, cabin or camper for heating purposes?

Yes No 13. Have you had a reliable mechanic check the exhaust system of your car within the past year?

Yes No 14. Do you ever run your auto engine in the garage while the garage door is shut?

Yes No 15. Do you leave the door closed between your attached garage and your house when you run your car engine?

Yes No 16. Do you keep your windows slightly open while driving in heavy traffic, although you have an air conditioner?

Yes No 17. While driving your station wagon, do you lower the tailgate to get a greater flow of air in the car?

Yes No 18. When you are selecting gas equipment, do you buy only those items that carry the seal of a national testing agency, such as the American Gas Association or the Underwriters' Laboratory?

Yes No 19. Have you ever converted, or are you about to convert, a fuel burner from one fuel to another without having it done by an expert?

Yes No 20. As an overnight guest at motels or hotels that have heating units located in the room, do you read operating instructions or ask how such appliances operate?

Scoring

Give yourself one point for each correct answer. A score of 20 points indicates that you have taken the most precautions to prevent carbon monoxide poisoning. A score of less than 20 points indicates you may need to take action to prevent CO poisoning from some unknown sources.

Answers

1. YES A yearly checkup of all fuel-burning venting systems in the home is desirable.
2. YES A yearly checkup of all combustion appliances is suggested. In many areas, upon request, the gas company will provide this service.
3. YES All gas appliances must have adequate ventilation so that CO will not accumulate.
4. YES Chimney vents often become blocked by debris causing a buildup of CO They should be checked annually.
5. NO Often a makeshift patch can lead to an accumulation of CO, and therefore should be avoided.
6. NO In-room vent pipes should be on a slight incline as they go toward the exterior. This will reduce leaking of toxic gases in case the joints or pipes are improperly fitted.
7. NO Using a gas range for heating can result in the accumulation of CO.
8. NO An unusual odor from a gas refrigerator often is the result of defects within the cooling unit. Odorless CO also may be given off.
9. NO The use of barbecue grills indoors will quickly result in dangerous levels of CO.
10. NO Burning charcoal-whether black, red, gray or white-gives off CO.
11. NO Although catalytic heaters produce heat without flame, combustion is occurring that can cause the production of CO.
12. NO Using a gas camp stove for heating the home, cabin or camper call result in the accumulation of CO.
13. YES Small leaks in the exhaust system of a car can lead to an accumulation of CO in the interior.
14. NO CO can rapidly build up while your auto engine is operated in a closed garage. Never run your car in a garage unless the outside door is open to provide ventilation.
15. YES CO can easily escape from a garage through a connecting door that opens into the house, although the garage door is open. Doors connecting a garage and house should be kept closed when the auto is running.
16. YES Even with an air conditioner, CO can be drawn into a car while it is being driven slowly in heavy traffic. Therefore, windows should be slightly opened.
17. NO If the tailgate is open, be sure to open vents or windows to increase the flow of air in the car. If the tailgate window is open and the other windows or the vents are closed, CO from the exhaust will be drawn into the car.
18. YES Buy only equipment carrying the seal of a national testing agency; otherwise, one may get poorly designed equipment, which may soon result in the production of CO.
19. NO An expert is needed to make proper modifications and to evaluate the venting capabilities of your appliance.
20. YES Even with adequately designed and properly installed heating equipment, the improper operation of this equipment can result in its malfunctioning and lead to the production of CO. Therefore, be sure you understand the correct way to operate any fuel-burning appliance before using it.

Source: Centers for Disease Control and Prevention

Checkup on Health Insurance Choices: Which Type Is Right for You?

Directions

For each group, choose the statement A or B that best describes how you feel:

A. Having complete freedom to choose doctors and hospitals is the most important thing to me in a health plan, even if it costs more.
B. Holding down my costs is the most important thing to me, even if it means limiting some of my choices.

A. I travel a lot or have children that live away from me and we may need to see doctors in other parts of the country.
B. I do not travel a lot and almost all care for my family will be needed in our local area.

A. I don't mind a health insurance plan that includes filling out forms or keeping receipts and sending them in for payment.
B. I prefer not to fill out forms or keep receipts. I want most of my care covered without a lot of paperwork.

A. In addition to my premiums, I am willing to pay for the cost of routine and preventive care, such as office visits, checkups, and shots. I also like knowing that I can get an appointment for these services when I want one.
B. I want a health plan that includes routine and preventive care. I don't mind if I have to wait for these services to be scheduled for an available appointment with my doctor.

A. If I need to see a specialist, I probably will ask my doctor for a recommendation, but I want to decide whom to go to and when. I don't want to have to see my primary care doctor each time before I can see a specialist.
B. I don't mind if my primary care doctor must refer me to specialists. If my doctor doesn't think I need special services, that is fine with me.

If your answers are mostly A: You want to make your own health care choices, even if it costs you more and takes more paperwork. Fee-for-service may be the best plan for you.

If your answers are mostly B: You are willing to give up some choices to hold down your medical costs. You also want help in managing your care. Consider a health maintenance organization.

If your answers are some A's and some B's: You might want to look for a plan such as a preferred provider organization that combines some of the features of fee-for-service and a health maintenance organization.

The differences among fee-for-service plans, HMOs, and PPOs are not as clear-cut as they once were. Fee-for-service plans have adopted some activities used by HMOs and PPOs to control the use of medical services. And HMOs and PPOs are offering more freedom to choose doctors, the way fee-for-service plans do. By studying your health insurance options carefully, you will be able to pick the one that provides you with the coverage you need, no matter what it is called.

Source: December 1992. Agency for Health Care Policy and Research, Rockville, MD.

Choosing a Doctor

Directions

Follow each of the steps.

Step One: Make a List of Doctors

1. If you are in a managed care plan, check the plan's list of doctors first.
2. Ask doctors or other health professionals who work with doctors, such as hospital nurses.
3. Check the "Physician Select" service of the Web site of the American Medical Association. This can give you lists of doctors, by specialty, who practice near you. You can also check on training and board certification: http://www.ama-assn.org/aps/amahg.htm.
4. Call a doctor referral service at a hospital. But keep in mind that these services usually refer you to any of the doctors on the staff of that hospital. The services do not have information on the quality of care these doctors provide.
5. Some local medical societies offer lists of doctors who are members. Again, these lists do not have information on the quality of care these doctors provide.
6. Ask family, friends, neighbors, and co-workers.

Step Two: Write your list here.

Name: ______________________________ Telephone:_________________________
Name: ______________________________ Telephone:_________________________
Name: ______________________________ Telephone:_________________________

Step Three: Check on Quality

Once you have a list of doctors, there are several ways to check on their skills and knowledge, and the quality of care they provide:

7. Find out if a consumer or other group has rated doctors in the area where you live. Again you will want to find out how reliable the ratings are.
8. Information on doctors in some States is available on the Internet at http://www.docboard.org. This Web site is run by Administrators in Medicine-a group of State medical board directors.
9. The American Board of Medical Specialties (800-776-2378) can tell you if the doctor is board certified. "Certified" means that the doctor has completed a training program in a specialty and has passed an exam (board) to assess his or her knowledge, skills, and experience to provide quality patient care in that specialty.
10. Call the American Medical Association (AMA) at 800-665-2882 for information on training, specialties, and board certification about many licensed doctors in the United States. This information also can be found in "Physician Select" at AMA's Web site: http://www.ama-assn.org/aps/amahg.htm.

Step Four: Contact the Doctors' Offices

When you have found a few names of doctors you might want to try, call their offices. The first thing to find out is whether the doctor is covered by your health plan and is taking new patients. If the doctor is not covered by your plan, are you prepared to pay the extra costs?

Below are some questions you might want to ask the office manager or other staff. You may have some additional questions. Note that some of these items might have more to do with the health plan than with the doctor's office.

Things to find out from office staff:

Which hospitals does the doctor use?

Doctor A: ______________________________
Doctor B: ______________________________
Doctor C: ______________________________

What are the office hours (when is the doctor available and when can I speak to office staff)?

Doctor A: ______________________________
Doctor B: ______________________________
Doctor C: ______________________________

Does the doctor or someone else in the office speak the language that I am most comfortable speaking?

Doctor A: ______________________________
Doctor B: ______________________________
Doctor C: ______________________________

How many other doctors "cover" for the doctor when he or she is not available? Who are they?

Doctor A: ______________________________
Doctor B: ______________________________
Doctor C: ______________________________

How long does it usually take to get a routine appointment?

Doctor A: ______________________________
Doctor B: ______________________________
Doctor C: ______________________________

How long might I need to wait in the office before seeing the doctor?

Doctor A: ______________________________
Doctor B: ______________________________
Doctor C: ______________________________

What happens if I need to cancel an appointment? Will I have to pay for it anyway?

Doctor A: ____________________
Doctor B: ____________________
Doctor C: ____________________

Does the office send reminders about prevention tests-for example, Pap smears?

Doctor A: ____________________
Doctor B: ____________________
Doctor C: ____________________

What do I do if I need urgent care or have an emergency?

Doctor A: ____________________
Doctor B: ____________________
Doctor C: ____________________

Does the doctor (or a nurse or physician assistant) give advice over the phone for common medical problems?

Doctor A: ____________________
Doctor B: ____________________
Doctor C: ____________________

You may also want to talk briefly with the doctor by phone or in person. Ask if you are able to do this and if there is a charge.

Step Five: The next step is to schedule a visit with your top choice.

During that first visit you will learn a lot about just how easy it is to talk with the doctor. You will also find out how well the doctor might meet your medical needs.

Ask yourself: Did the doctor...

1. Give me a chance to ask questions?	YES NO
2. Really listen to my questions?	YES NO
3. Answer in terms I understood?	YES NO
4. Show respect for me?	YES NO
5. Ask me questions?	YES NO
6. Make me feel comfortable?	YES NO
7. Address the health problem(s) I came with?	YES NO
8. Ask me my preferences about different kinds of treatments?	YES NO
9. Spend enough time with me?	YES NO

Scoring

Trust your own reactions when deciding whether this doctor is the right one for you. But you also may want to give the relationship some time to develop. It takes more than one visit for you and your doctor to get to know each other.

Source: Choosing a Doctor. Your Guide to Choosing Quality Health Care. December 1998, Agency for Health Care Policy and Research, Rockville, MD.

Making Decisions About Surgery

Some surgery has to be done right away. But most surgery is not an emergency. That means you have time to talk with your doctor and decide what is best for you. Here are some questions you may want to ask your doctor or surgeon.

1. Do I really need this surgery? Is there some other way to treat my condition?

2. What will happen if I wait until later to have surgery? Or never have it at all?

3. Where will the surgery be performed?

4. Does the surgeon, hospital or surgery center have a lot of experience with this kind of procedure?

5. Is the surgeon experienced and qualified to perform surgery?

6. What complications or side effects might I have?

7. What kind of pain might I have? How will it be treated?

8. How long will it take me to recover? Will I need help at home? What kind of help?

9. How much does surgery cost?

10. Will my health plan pay?

Source: Choosing Treatments, Your Guide To Choosing Quality Health Care, December 1998. Agency for Health Care Policy and Research, Rockville, MD.

Choosing a Health Plan

Directions

The next section lists several questions you may want to consider when choosing a health plan. These questions are based on research about what consumers want to know when choosing health plans. Under each question you will find more information to help you choose the plan that is right for you. You also will find a way to compare the health plans you are looking at. Here's how:

Space is provided for comparing three plans. Enter the name of each plan on a separate line.

Plan A: ______________________________
Plan B: ______________________________
Plan C: ______________________________

Read the questions. Which are most important to you in choosing a health plan?

* Do members rate the plan highly on things that are important to me?
* Does the plan provide preventive services to help keep people well?
* Does it do a good job of helping them get better when they are sick?
* Is the plan accredited?
* Does the plan have the doctors and hospitals I want or need?
* Does the plan provide the benefits I need?
* Do the doctors, pharmacies, and other services in the plan have convenient times and locations?
* Does the plan meet my budget?

Read and think about the information under each question. Then ask yourself the question. If the answer is "yes" for a plan, check the box next to its name. Of course, the answers to these questions may not be as simple as "yes" or "no." Still, these questions should help you to think about and compare your health plan choices. Do this for all the questions you have chosen.

Rate Your Health Plan Choices

Do members rate the plan highly on things that are important to me?

Plan A: [ ] Yes
Plan B: [ ] Yes
Plan C: [ ] Yes

Does the plan provide preventive services to help keep people well?

Plan A: [ ] Yes
Plan B: [ ] Yes
Plan C: [ ] Yes

Does it do a good job of helping them get better when they are sick?

Plan A: [ ] Yes
Plan B: [ ] Yes
Plan C: [ ] Yes

Is the plan accredited?

Plan A: [ ] Yes
Plan B: [ ] Yes
Plan C: [ ] Yes

The Joint Commission on Accreditation of Healthcare Organizations (JCAHO) evaluates and accredits all types of health care organizations. Visit the JCAHO Web site: http://www.jcaho.org. Information on accredited organizations is free of charge.

Does the plan have the doctors and hospitals I want or need?

Plan A: [ ] Yes
Plan B: [ ] Yes
Plan C: [ ] Yes

Does the plan provide the benefits I need?

Plan A: [ ] Yes
Plan B: [ ] Yes
Plan C: [ ] Yes

Do the doctors, pharmacies, and other services in the plan have convenient times and locations?

Plan A: [ ] Yes
Plan B: [ ] Yes
Plan C: [ ] Yes

Does the plan meet my budget?

Plan A: [ ] Yes
Plan B: [ ] Yes
Plan C: [ ] Yes

Use the health plan materials from your employer or the plans to answer these questions and enter the information on the line provided under each plan.

Cost	Plan A	Plan B	Plan C
How much will the premium cost me each month?	_______	_______	_______
If there is a deductible, how much will I have to pay before the plan starts to pay for medical care?	_______	_______	_______

For prescription medicines? _______ _______ _______

How much will I have to pay (co-payment) each time I use a service?
Doctor visit _______ _______ _______
Hospital visit _______ _______ _______
Prescription _______ _______ _______

How much more will I need to pay if I go outside the health plan's network of doctors, hospitals, and other providers to get services? _______ _______ _______

Source: Choosing a Health Plan. Your Guide to Choosing Quality Health Care, December 1998. Agency for Health Care Policy and Research, Rockville, MD

Choosing Treatments

Directions

The first step in getting the right treatment is to tell your doctor what's going on. This information might include:

Your symptoms: ____________________

When they first started: ____________________

When they occur: ____________________

Are they getting better? Worse? ____________________

What makes them better? Worse? ____________________

Are they affecting eating, sleeping, or other activities? How?

____

Medicines you take: ____________________

Before a treatment decision is made, your doctor needs to make a diagnosis. Medical tests are an important way to help your doctor learn about the problem. It is important to make sure that any tests your doctor suggests are appropriate for you.

Medical Tests

Doctors order blood tests, x-rays, and other tests to help diagnose medical problems. Perhaps you do not know why you need a particular test or you don't understand how it will help you. Here are some questions to ask:

How is the test done? ____________________

What kind of information will the test provide?

____

Is this test the only way to find out that information?

____

What are the benefits and risks of having this test?

____

How accurate is the test? ____________________

What do I need to do to prepare for the test? (What you do or don't do may affect the accuracy of the test results.)

____

Will the test be uncomfortable? ______________________________

How long will it take to get the results, and how will I get them?

____

What's the next step after the test? ______________________________

What about the test results?

* Do not assume that no news is good news. If you do not hear from your doctor, call to get your test results.
* If you and your doctor think the test results may not be right, have the test done again.

Getting the Diagnosis

When your doctor has decided what your problem is, he or she will give you a diagnosis. But you should know that reaching a diagnosis can be hard. Sometimes it can take a long time. And sometimes it is hard to find out exactly what is wrong. Ask your doctor to explain what you have and how it might affect you and your family.

What is the diagnosis? ______________________________

What is my prognosis (outlook for the future)?

____

What changes, if any, will I need to make in my daily life?

____

Is there a chance that someone else in my family might get the same condition?

____

Will I need special help at home for my condition? If so, what type of help?

____

Looking at the Options

The next step is for you and your doctor to look at your treatment options. Your doctor may recommend one or more of the following:

* Behavior change (for example: eating a healthier diet, getting more exercise, quitting smoking).
* Prescription medicine.
* Non-prescription ("over-the-counter") medicines.
* Surgery.
* Rehabilitation (such as physical therapy).
* Other treatments (for example, chiropractic services, massage, or acupuncture).
* "Watchful waiting." (You and your doctor keep track of your symptoms and watch for any changes. If there are changes, then treatment might be the next step.)

What is the recommended treatment? Are there other choices?

____

What are the chances the treatment will work?

____

What are the expected results? When will I see them?

____

What are the risks? ____

What are the benefits? ____

Are there any side effects? (Most treatments have them.) What can be done about them?

____

Is the treatment painful? How can the pain be controlled?

____

What happens if I choose to have no treatment at all?

____

How much does the treatment cost? Will my health plan pay?

____

Once you have the answers to these questions, you might want to make a chart of "Benefits and Risks" or "Pros and Cons" to help you decide if the treatment is right for you. Here is a sample chart:

Benefits (Pros)	Risks (Cons)
* Treatment has worked well for others with my condition.	* Some minor side effects (rash, stomach upset) could be troubling.
* The medicine only needs to be taken once a day.	* The medicine is costly.
* No major side effects are expected.	

Source: Choosing Treatments. Your Guide to Choosing Quality Health Care. December 1998. Agency for Health Care Policy and Research, Rockville, MD.

Review and Practice Tests

By Lynne Blesz Vestal

1 Promoting Healthy Behavior Change

General Review Questions

1. What are the major dimensions of health?
2. Define prevention and list the three forms of prevention.
3. What are the major factors that influence behavior and behavior-change decisions?
4. According to the Health Belief Model, what factors must support a belief in order for a change to be likely to occur?
5. What are the components for analyzing a behavior you want to change?

Practice Test #1

1. Prior to the 1800s, poor health was often associated with
   a. the lack of penicillin.
   b. the lack of medical care.
   c. poor hygiene and unsanitary conditions.
   d. diseases of heart and circulatory system.

2. The eradication of smallpox and the control of rubella are both due to which achievement in public health?
   a. control of infectious diseases
   b. safe and healthy foods
   c. maternal and infant care
   d. vaccinations

3. Intolerance aimed at people who fail to meet our own expectations of health defines
   a. health bashing.
   b. health deficiency.
   c. health fixation.
   d. wellness fixation.

4. Learning specific behaviors by watching others perform them is called
   a. shaping.
   b. modeling.
   c. imagined rehearsal.
   d. situational inducement.

5. What is the leading cause of death for all 15 to 24-year-olds in the United States?
   a. cancer
   b. accidents and adverse effects
   c. stroke
   d. heart disease

6. According to researchers at the Harvard School of Public Health and the World Health Organization, which of the following will increase as a major threat to health over the next two decades?
   a. tuberculosis
   b. diarrheal diseases
   c. congenital abnormalities
   d. ischemic heart disease

7. An appraisal of the relationship between some object, action, or idea and some attribute of that object, action or idea, is called a(n)
   a. attitude.
   b. cue to action.
   c. predisposing factor.
   d. belief.

8. Life experiences, knowledge, cultural and ethnic inheritance, and cultural beliefs and values are
   a. predisposing factors.
   b. enabling factors.
   c. readiness factors.
   d. reinforcing factors.

9. Attending a health education seminar ton quitting cigarette smoking is an example of
   a. primary prevention.
   b. health promotion.
   c. secondary prevention.
   d. tertiary prevention.

10. The number of existing cases of a disease or disability defines
    a. prevalence.
    b. incidence.
    c. health status.
    d. cumulative percentage.

11. What type of reinforcers include such things as loving looks, affectionate hugs, and praise?
a. consumable reinforcers
b. activity reinforcers
c. manipulative reinforcers
d. social reinforcers

12. Taking prevention steps that stop a health problem before it starts is called
a. primary prevention.
b. secondary prevention.
c. wellness.
d. health promotion.

13. What is the state of being that precedes a behavioral change?
a. cue to action
b. readiness
c. values
d. locus of control

14. Using positive self-affirmations to promote positive self-esteem and behaviors is a form of
a. thought stopping.
b. cues to action.
c. modeling.
d. self-talk.

15. The setting events for a behavior that cue or stimulate a person to act in certain ways are called
a. antecedents.
b. frequency of events.
c. consequences.
d. cues to action.

Practice Test #2

1. In developing regions of the world, infectious disease and malnutrition are being replaced as the leading causes of disability and death by
a. depression and heart disease.
b. war.
c. self-inflicted injuries.
d. measles.

2. Starting off by walking a mile a day so that eventually you will be able to run 3 miles a day is an example of which behavior change technique?
a. shaping
b. visualization
c. modeling
d. reinforcement

3. What stage of change characterizes a person who is in denial and has no intention of taking any action?
a. precontemplation
b. preparation
c. contemplation
d. maintenance

4. Age, gender, race and ethnic background are all
a. sociopsychological variables.
b. psychological variables.
c. demographic variables.
d. structural variables.

5. The key behaviors that will help people live longer include
a. maintaining healthy eating habits.
b. sleeping a minimum of seven hours.
c. weight management.
d. All of the above

6. Our ability to think clearly, reason objectively, and use one's "brain power" effectively to meet life's challenges is defined as
a. social health.
b. intellectual health.
c. emotional health.
d. spiritual health.

7. The number of new cases of a disease or disability is called
a. prevalence.
b. incidence.
c. health status.
d. cumulative percentage.

8. An academically trained health educator who has passed a national competency examination for prevention/intervention programming is a
a. primary prevention specialist.
b. health promotion specialist.
c. certified health education specialist.
d. certified prevention specialist.

9. What dimension of health refers to the ability to have satisfying interpersonal relationships?
   a. spiritual health
   b. emotional health
   c. social health
   d. mental health

10. What theory proposes that our behaviors result from our intentions to perform actions?
    a. social learning theory
    b. modeling
    c. cues to action
    d. theory of reasoned action

11. Which of the following is *not* a factor in influencing behavior and behavior-change decisions?
    a. circumstantial factors
    b. enabling factors
    c. reinforcing factors
    d. predisposing factors

12. You want to bicycle for exercise but do not have access to a bicycle. This is an example of
    a. predisposing factors.
    b. enabling factors.
    c. reinforcing factors.
    d. cues to action.

13. A relatively stable set of beliefs, feelings, and behavioral tendencies in relation to something or someone is called a(n)
    a. belief.
    b. value.
    c. social environment.
    d. attitude.

14. Delicious edibles such as candy, cookies, or gourmet meals are examples of
    a. consumable reinforcers.
    b. activity reinforcers.
    c. extrinsic rewards.
    d. manipulative reinforcers.

15. What form of cognitive therapy is based on the premise that there is a close connection between what people say to themselves and how they feel?
    a. theory of reasoned action
    b. thought blocking
    c. locus of control
    d. rational-emotive therapy

2 Psychosocial Health

General Review Questions

1. What are the basic elements shared by psychologically healthy people?
2. What are the traditional forms of therapy?
3. What internal factors shape psychological well-being?
4. List the risk factors for suicide.
5. What are ways to develop and maintain self-esteem?

Practice Test #1

1. The "feeling" part of psychosocial health that includes your emotional reactions to life is called
   a. emotional health.
   b. social health.
   c. spiritual health.
   d. self-esteem.

2. What disorder is believed to be caused by a malfunction in the hypothalamus?
   a. schizophrenia
   b. major depression
   c. seasonal affective disorder
   d. generalized anxiety disorder

3. Mary Jo cannot go to bed until she has checked and rechecked all the windows in the house to make sure they are shut. This behavior is an example of a(n)
   a. phobia.
   b. panic attack.
   c. obession.
   d. compulsion.

4. "Free-floating anxiety" is a distinguishing feature of
   a. panic attacks.
   b. social phobias.
   c. obsessive-compulsive disorder.
   d. generalized anxiety disorder.

5. What is the most common phobic response?
   a. social phobia
   b. claustrophobia
   c. xenophobia
   d. acrophobia

6. What are the two most common psychotherapeutic therapies for depression?
   a. psychodynamic and Gestalt
   b. humanistic and Gestalt
   c. cognitive therapy and interpersonal therapy
   d. behavior and family

7. A mentally healthy student who receives a D on an exam may be very disappointed by her grade and will
   a. reassess her course options and withdraw from the course.
   b. try to assess the reasons she did poorly.
   c. make an appointment with the instructor to try to get her grade changed.
   d. become cynical about passing the course and give up trying to do her best.

8. Belief in some unifying force that gives a sense of purpose or meaning to life is called
   a. mental health.
   b. psychological health.
   c. spiritual health.
   d. egocentric health.

9. Strong social bonds function to
   a. provide intimacy.
   b. provide opportunities for giving or receiving nurturance.
   c. provide reassurance of one's worth.
   d. All of the above

10. A complex interaction of one's mental, emotional, social, and spiritual health is known as
   a. wellness.
   b. psychosocial health.
   c. health promotion.
   d. psychosocial prevention.

11. A psychologically unhealthy person is characterized by all of the following, *except*
    a. laughs, usually at others.
    b. high energy, resilient, and enjoys challenges.
    c. has little fun, no time for him- or herself.
    d. has serious bouts of depression.

12. A negative evaluation of an entire group of people that is typically based on unfavorable ideas about the group is called
    a. personal control.
    b. prejudice.
    c. phobia.
    d. learned helplessness.

13. Our family, the greater environment, and social supports/social bonds are examples of
    a. internal factors.
    b. external factors.
    c. intrinsic factors.
    d. self-efficacy.

14. Marty flunked a math class two times and does not believe that he is good at math. He has resolved himself to not being able to graduate because he will never pass a required math class. This is known as
    a. learned helplessness.
    b. external locus of control.
    c. seasonal affective disorder.
    d. post-traumatic shock syndrome.

15. A person with a Ph.D. degree and training in psychology, is called a
    a. psychiatrist.
    b. psychologist.
    c. social worker.
    d. psychoanalyst.

Practice Test #2

1. Susie is worried about the clothes she wears and says that she needs to buy a car that projects her as successful. What stage of Jung's View of Personal Growth and Spiritual Development is she experiencing?
    a. the dawn of life
    b. the morning of life
    c. the noon of life
    d. the evening of life

2. Sam is fatigued and is sleeping too much. He has no interest in hanging out with his friends or family. In addition, he no longer cares to snowboard or participate in other hobbies. Sam may be experiencing
    a. anxiety.
    b. a phobia.
    c. depression.
    d. posttraumatic stress disorder.

3. What is the basic assumption of humanistic therapy?
    a. People are good and have innate worth.
    b. Behavior is motivated by both unconscious forces and interpersonal experiences.
    c. Problems in relationships entail everybody involved in them.
    d. Behavior is largely controlled by environmental contingencies.

4. The most common onset for schizophrenia is in
    a. early childhood.
    b. late adolescence.
    c. middle adulthood.
    d. late adulthood.

5. What is the most common psychiatric disorder in the United States?
    a. schizophrenia
    b. major depression
    c. generalized anxiety disorder
    d. bipolar disorder

6. Which of the following is *not* a component of subjective-well-being?
    a. satisfaction with present life
    b. mindfulness practice
    c. relative presence of positive emotions
    d. relative absence of negative emotions

7. Sleep apnea is typically caused by
    a. excessive amounts of the hormone melatonin.
    b. high levels of stress.
    c. high blood pressure.
    d. upper respiratory tract problems.

8. Continual failure that causes people to give up and fail to take any action to help themselves is called
   a. learned helplessness.
   b. protective factors.
   c. learned failure.
   d. learned survival.

9. One's sense of self-respect or self-confidence refers to
   a. self-esteem.
   b. social support.
   c. ego.
   d. developmental capabilities.

10. All of the following are warnings of suicide, *except*
    a. a preoccupation with themes of death.
    b. increased interest in classes or work.
    c. failure to recover from a personal loss or crisis.
    d. giving away prized possessions.

11. Which of the following is *not* true about phobias?
    a. They tend to be more prevalent in men than in women.
    b. They are deep and persistent fears of specific objects, activities, or situations.
    c. Simple phobias may be treated successfully with behavioral therapy.
    d. Social phobias may require more extensive therapy.

12. A psychological disorder among women that is characterized by depression, irritability, and other symptoms of increased stress is called
    a. depression.
    b. phobia.
    c. premenstrual syndrome depression.
    d. panic attack.

13. A medical doctor who specializes in treating emotional disorders is a(n)
    a. oncologist.
    b. psychoanalyst.
    c. psychologist.
    d. psychiatrist.

14. Therapy that aims to help a patient look at life rationally and to correct habitually pessimistic thought patterns is called
    a. family therapy.
    b. psychodynamic therapy.
    c. cognitive therapy.
    d. behavioral therapy.

15. Suicide is more likely to occur among
    a. college students.
    b. high school dropouts.
    c. high school students.
    d. middle-age males.

3 Managing Stress

General Review Questions

1. List the phases of Selye's General Adaptation Syndrome.
2. What are the sources of both eustress and distress?
3. Distinguish between two stress-related personality types: Type A and Type B.
4. Describe the characteristics of psychological hardiness.
5. Describe stress inoculation.

Practice Test #1

1. Psychologically healthy people are characterized by all of the following, *except*
   a. control.
   b. challenge.
   c. changing.
   d. commitment.

2. When the hypothalamus perceives that extra energy is needed to fight a stressor, it stimulates the adrenal glands to release the hormone
   a. melatonin.
   b. epinephrine.
   c. serotonin.
   d. cortisol.

3. Stress that presents positive opportunities for personal growth is called
   a. homeostasis.
   b. strain.
   c. eustress.
   d. distress.

4. What did a Harvard study conclude is the most important predictor of physical health?
   a. age
   b. gender
   c. mental health
   d. socioeconomic status

5. Jack is an air-traffic controller who works under high-pressure at one of the busiest airports in the nation. Under excessive stress daily, Jack is at risk for experiencing
   a. burnout.
   b. eustress.
   c. conflict.
   d. overload.

6. Patty feels she doesn't have any control over events in her life, such as the type of job she will get after graduating from college or where she will live. Patty has an:
   a. internal locus of control and low self-efficacy.
   b. internal locus of control and high self-efficacy.
   c. external locus of control and low self-efficacy.
   d. external locus of control and high self-efficacy.

7. Studies of traditional and nontraditional students find that
   a. nontraditional students have more time contraints than traditional students.
   b. nontraditional students experience more academic stress than traditional students.
   c. nontraditional students report less satisfaction in schiool than traditional students.
   d. nontraditional students experience more health problems than traditional students.

8. What branch of the autonomic nervous system is responsible for energizing the body for either fight or flight?
   a. central nervous system
   b. parasympathetic nervous system
   c. sympathetic nervous system
   d. endocrine system

9. What key region of the brain is responsible for controlling the sympathetic nervous system and directing the stress response?
   a. pituitary gland
   b. hypothalamus
   c. adrenal glands
   d. adrenal cortex

10. The phase of the general adaptation syndrome in which the physical and psychological energy used to fight the stressors have been depleted is called the
   a. alarm phase.
   b. resistance phase.
   c. endurance phase.
   d. exhaustion phase.

11. Conflict occurs when we
   a. are forced to face two incompatible demands, opportunities, needs, or goals.
   b. are forced to speed up, intensify or shift the direction of our performance.
   c. must make adjustments to change.
   d. None of the above

12. The wear and tear that our bodies and minds sustain during the process of adjusting to or resisting a stressor is called
   a. strain.
   b. eustress.
   c. stress.
   d. resistance.

13. During the alarm phase of the general adaptation syndrome, the
   a. stressor disturbs homeostasis.
   b. body reacts to the stressor and adjusts to allow the system to return to homeostasis
   c. body's adaptation energy stores. release cells for energy and renew the energy reserves.
   d. energy stores are depleted and the organism dies.

14. Mood-elevating, pain-killing chemicals that have a morphinelike action on the body and are produced by exercise are called
   a. endorphins.
   b. adrenaline.
   c. cortisol.
   d. norepinephrine.

15. An area of scientific investigation that analyzes the relationship between the mind's response to stress and the ability of the immune system to function effectively is called
   a. psychoneuroimmunology.
   b. adaptation.
   c. resistance.
   d. immunocompetence.

Practice Test #2

1. The adaptive response to stress occurs when
   a. the body attempts to return to homeostasis.
   b. the stressor is no longer present.
   c. there is a sense of relief that survival has been achieved.
   d. resistance to the stress has adjusted to a positive result.

2. In a large study of chronic stressors, male and female college students differed significantly in the things they perceived to be significant stressors. Which of the following do women identify as a frequent stressor?
   a. not enough friends
   b. concerns about alcohol use
   c. not having someone to date
   d. having an overload of school work

3. What is the final phase of the general adaptation syndrome?
   a. alarm
   b. exhaustion
   c. resistance
   d. overload

4. Following a shooting that left two students dead, the students who witnessed the murder may suffer from
   a. panic attacks.
   b. obsessive-compulsive disorder.
   c. generalized anxiety disorder.
   d. posttraumatic stress disorder.

5. Events that can result in debilitative stress or strain are known as
   a. strain.
   b. stress.
   c. distress.
   d. adjustment.

6. A balanced physical state in which all of the body's systems function smoothly results in
   a. homeostasis.
   b. distress.
   c. eustress.
   d. general adaptation syndrome.

7. The pituitary hormone that signals the adrenal glands to release cortisol is
   a. epinephrine.
   b. adrenocorticotropic hormone.
   c. endorphin.
   d. adrenaline.

8. Feeling forced to speed up, intensify, or shift the direction of your behavior to meet a higher standard of performance, can result in
   a. hassles.
   b. pressure.
   c. change.
   d. conflict.

9. A state of physical and mental exhaustion caused by excessive stress is called
   a. conflict.
   b. overload.
   c. hassles.
   d. burnout.

10. Overcrowding, discrimination, unemployment, inflation, and poverty are examples of
    a. burnout.
    b. conflict.
    c. psychosocial stress.
    d. background distressors.

11. The part of the autonomic nervous system that functions to slow all the systems stimulated by the stress response is called the
    a. parasympathetic nervous system.
    b. sympathetic nervous system.
    c. central nervous system.
    d. cerebral cortex.

12. Preliminary research data on stress levels and immune functioning supports that during periods of prolonged stress, elevated adrenal hormones
    a. destroy or reduce the ability of natural killer-T cells to aid the immune response.
    b. improve the ability of natural killer-T cells to aid the immune response.
    c. have no known affect on natural killer-T cells to aid the immune response.
    d. None of the above

13. A conscious attempt to simplify life in an effort to reduce the stresses and strains of modern living is called
    a. adaptation.
    b. conflict resolution.
    c. burnout reduction.
    d. downshifting.

14. What stress management technique involves self-monitoring by machine of physical responses to stress and attempts to subsequently control these responses?
    a. meditation
    b. biofeedback
    c. hypnosis
    d. deep-muscle relaxation

15. Losing your keys or having the grocery bag rip on the way to the door are examples of
    a. pressure.
    b. incongruent goals and behaviors.
    c. hassles.
    d. conflict.

4 Violence and Abuse

General Review Questions

1. List the phases of Lenore Walker's cycle of violence.
2. Describe the factors that increase the likelihood of violent acts.
3. What are the most important assumptions in our society that prevent the realization of the true nature of sexual assault.
4. What causes young people to join gangs?
5. What preventive actions can be taken to ensure that sexual harassment will not be repeated?

Practice Test #1

1. What type of program should elementary schools use to prevent gang membership?
   a. Programs that focus on the short-term consequences of gang membership.
   b. Programs that focus on the long-term consequences of gang membership.
   c. Programs that focus at an early age on reducing alienation from family, friends, and school.
   d. Programs that focus at an early age on the illegal actions of gang members.

2. What is the single most identifiable risk factor for predicting child abuse?
   a. spouse abuse
   b. low socioeconomic status
   c. unemplyment
   d. previous juvenile record

3. What is the correct sequence of the cycle of violence theory?
   a. remorse/reconciliation, acute battering, tension building
   b. tension building, acute battering, remorse/reconciliation
   c. tension building, remorse/reconciliation, acute battering
   d. remorse/reconciliation, acute battering, tension building

4. Kurt and Brenda are in a violent relationship. After Kurt struck Brenda, she tried to be more pleasing and tried to anticipate Kurt's needs in order to forestall another beating, assuming guilt for doing something to provoke him. Which phase of the cycle of violence are they in?
   a. acute battering
   b. chronic battering
   c. remorse/reconciliation
   d. tension building

5. A group of students were discussing a recently publicized sexual assault. One student comments that some women dress too provocatively. What social assumption has this student made?
   a. minimization
   b. trivialization
   c. blaming the victim
   d. "boys will be boys"

6. A set of behaviors that produces injuries, regardless of whether they are intentional or unintentional is called
   a. aggression.
   b. accidents.
   c. abuse.
   d. violence.

7. The threat of abuse and violence, including slapping, shoving, or breaking bones by someone in the home environment, is called
   a. rape.
   b. sexual assault.
   c. domestic assault.
   d. domestic violence.

8. What is the single greatest cause of injury to women?
   a. auto accidents
   b. rape
   c. domestic violence
   d. muggings

9. Child abusers tend to
   a. have been abused as a child.
   b. have feelings of isolation.
   c. have a tendency to abuse alcohol and/or drugs.
   d. All of the above

10. The most frequent sexual abusers of children are
   a. grandfathers.
   b. siblings or cousings.
   c. older friends.
   d. child's parents, parents' companions, or spouses of the child's parents.

11. Acquaintance or date rape is most common among
   a. minority high school females.
   b. college women.
   c. mothers with small children.
   d. women in professional jobs.

12. Rape by one person known to the victim and that does not involve a physical beating or use of a weapon is called
   a. simple assault.
   b. sexual assault.
   c. simple rape.
   d. aggravated rape.

13. Any act in which one person is sexually intimate with another without the other's consent defines
   a. sexual assault.
   b. sexual abuse.
   c. rape.
   d. sexual harassment.

14. Injuries that occur without anyone planning or intending that harm occur are called
   a. assaults.
   b. intentional injuries.
   c. unintentional injuries.
   d. circumstantial injuries.

15. Killing someone in self-defense is classified as what type of homicide?
   a. second-degree murder
   b. involuntary manslaughter
   c. justifiable homicide
   d. misdemeanor manslaughter

Practice Test #2

1. Aggression that is part of an emotional reaction brought about by frustrating life-experiences is called
   a. violence.
   b. primary aggression.
   c. domestic violence.
   d. reactive aggression.

2. Which phase of the cycle of violence is also known as the honeymoon?
   a. acute battering
   b. tension building
   c. remorse/reconciliation
   d. chronic battering

3. The assumption that men just cannot control themselves once they are aroused defines which social contributor to sexual assault?
   a. minimization
   b. blaming the victim
   c. "boys will be boys"
   d. female masochism

4. For the average American, the lifetime probability of being murdered is
   a. 1 in 450
   b. 1 in 153
   c. 1 in 28
   d. 1 in 3

5. Hate crimes tend to be characteristically
   a. excessively brutal.
   b. perpetrated at random on total strangers.
   c. perpetrated by multiple offenders.
   d. All of the above

6. Risk factors for gang membership include all of the following, *except*
   a. high self-esteem.
   b. history of family violence.
   c. living in gang-controlled neighborhoods.
   d. academic problems.

7. To reduce the risk of personal assaults while on the street, a person should
   a. walk with others.
   b. at night, avoid dark parking lots, wooded areas, and any place that offers an assailant good cover.
   c. carry change to make a phone call.
   d. All of the above

8. Rape that involves multiple attackers, strangers, weapons, or a physical beating is called
   a. sexual assault.
   b. simple rape.
   c. aggravated rape.
   d. simple assault.

9. Date rape is a(n)
   a. miscommunication between two individuals.
   b. act of violence.
   c. misperception on the part of males.
   d. inconsistent message that women give to men.

10. Violence that is directed randomly at persons affiliated with a particular group and is based on prejudice and discrimination is called
   a. physical abuse.
   b. psychological violence.
   c. social abuse.
   d. ethnoviolence.

11. A gang of white youth has as its sole purpose to commit acts of hatred toward any ethnic groups in their neighborhood. Their behavior reflects
   a. primary aggression.
   b. secondary aggression.
   c. reactive aggression.
   d. proactive aggression.

12. What is the leading cause of death among black males aged 15 to 34?
   a. cancer
   b. suicide
   c. homicide
   d. auto accidents

13. When Susan met with her boss, he told her that she looked very attractive in the dress she was wearing. Susan took offense to his remark. His comment constitutes
   a. sexual abuse.
   b. simple rape.
   c. sexual harassment.
   d. simple assault.

14. Homicide with malicious intent but without premeditation is classified as
   a. first-degree murder.
   b. second-degree murder.
   c. felony-murder.
   d. voluntary manslaughter.

15. Lenore Walker developed a theory of
   a. hate crimes.
   b. violence.
   c. sexual harassment.
   d. sexual abuse of children.

5 Healthy Relationships

General Review Questions

1. What psychological needs do intimate relationships fulfill?
2. Describe the characteristics of intimate sexual relationships.
3. List the characteristics of a dysfunctional family.
4. What are the causes of jealousy?
5. Discuss the reasons for divorce.

Practice Test #1

1. Intimate relationships are characterized by all of the following, *except*
   a. behavioral interdependence.
   b. need fulfillment.
   c. financial commitment.
   d. emotional attachment.

2. Experts tend to describe communication as
   a. the symbolic process of shared meanings.
   b. talking and listening.
   c. sending messages with words or your body.
   d. the process of using a common language to exchange information.

3. Roberto defines himself as a student, a young Republican and a Mexican-American. This is an example of
   a. self-motivation.
   b. self-concept.
   c. self-esteem.
   d. self-knowledge.

4. Psychologist Carl Rogers believed that weak relationships were characterized by
   a. inhibited self-disclosure.
   b. repressed self-esteem.
   c. untapped self-concept.
   d. unexpressed self-knowledge.

5. Assertive communicators are people who get their points across while at the same time
   a. making listeners feel intimidated.
   b. revealing their timid nature.
   c. making listeners on the defensive.
   d. respecting the rights of others.

6. According to McAdams, most people are fortunate to develop _________ lasting friendships in a lifetime.
   a. one or two
   b. two or four
   c. four or five
   d. five or seven

7. The type of family that includes unrelated people living together for ideological, economic, or other reasons, is a(n)
   a. communal family.
   b. polygamous family.
   c. extended family.
   d. family of origin.

8. Friendships are characterized by all of the following, *except*
   a. prearranged roles.
   b. respect.
   c. confiding.
   d. acceptance.

9. According to the Sternberg's triangular theory of love, which of the following is *not* a key ingredient of love?
   a. intimacy
   b. infatuation
   c. passion
   d. Ddecision/commitment

10. Regardless of the form or structure of families, the one unique characteristic that is common is
    a. shared finances.
    b. shared cultural practices.
    c. societally approved structure.
    d. the special caring, regard, and bonding that a group of people having shared interests has for each other.

11. What percentage of all Americans marry at least once?
    a. 35%
    b. 50%
    c. 75%
    d. 90%

12. The only available relationship option for lesbian and gay couples is
    a. open-relationship marriage.
    b. cohabitation.
    c. common-law marriage.
    d. polygamy.

13. Divorce rates are highest among people
    a. Below 30 years of age.
    b. 30-40 years of age.
    c. 40-50 years of age.
    d. 65 years or older.

14. To maintain a good relationship, self-nurturance involves
    a. being responsible for one's own decisions and actions.
    b. maintaining a balance of sleeping, eating, exercising, working, relaxing, and socializing.
    c. learning from one's bad choices.
    d. All of the above

15. Breakdowns in relationships usually begin with
    a. unresolved conflicts over money.
    b. changes in communication.
    c. sexual difficulties.
    d. spending time apart.

Practice Test #2

1. The ability to give to and receive from others emotionally without fear is called
    a. behavioral interdependence.
    b. need fulfillment.
    c. emotional availability.
    d. emotional attachment.

2. *Family of origin* refers to
    a. the people present in the household during the child's first few years of life.
    b. a child's parents and their offspring.
    c. a child's parents.
    d. all of a child's ancestors.

3. Turner and Rubinson concluded that friends share experiences and feelings with each other that they don't share with other people. This characteristic is referred to as
    a. enjoyment.
    b. respect.
    c. spontaneity.
    d. confiding.

4. "Alexithymia" refers to the
    a. inability to actively identify and communicate feelings.
    b. process of revealing one's inner thoughts and feelings to another person.
    c. dialect or speech patterns of each gender.
    d. aversive reaction evoked by a real or imagined relationship involving a person's partner and a third person.

5. The mutual impact that people have on each other as their lives and daily activities become intertwined is called
    a. need fulfillment.
    b. social integration.
    c. assistance.
    d. behavioral interdependence.

6. Close relationships with another person in which you offer and are offered validation, understanding, and a sense of being valued intellectually, emotionally, and physically are called
    a. friendships.
    b. intimate relationships.
    c. need fulfillment.
    d. nurturing relationships.

7. The skills needed for developing friendships include all of the following, *except*
    a. self-disclosure.
    b. negotiation.
    c. compromise.
    d. intimidation.

8. According to Fisher, attraction and falling in love follow a predictable pattern based on
    a. imprinting.
    b. attraction.
    c. attachment.
    d. All of the above

9. In comparison to friendship, love relationships are characterized by all of the following, *except*
    a. fascination.
    b. sexual desire.
    c. mutual assistance.
    d. giving the utmost.

10. Which of the following best describes the differences between men and women in selecting partners?
    a. Men are more likely than women to select their partners on the basis of youth and physical attractiveness.
    b. Women are more likely to select partners who are opposite of themselves in attitudes and values.
    c. Women are more likely than men to select their partners on the basis of youth and physical attractiveness.
    d. Men are more likely than women to place greater emphasis on financial prospects.

11. Which of the following factors are important when choosing a partner?
    a. proximity
    b. similarities
    c. reciprocity
    d. All of the above

12. Of those people who divorce, nearly ____ percent will remarry.
    a. 30
    b. 55
    c. 67
    d. 80

13. Although physical attractiveness is an important criterion for women in mate selection, they place a greater emphasis on partners who
    a. are at least five years younger.
    b. have good financial prospects.
    c. maintain strong family ties, especially with their mothers.
    d. possess athletic prowess.

14. Developing individual potential through a balanced and realistic appreciation of self-worth and ability is known as
    a. accountability.
    b. self-nurturance.
    c. trust.
    d. mutuality.

15. The median age for first marriages is
    a. 23.3 years for males; 21.6 years for females.
    b. 26.3 years for males; 24.0 years for females.
    c. 26.1 years for males; 23.9 years for females.
    d. 27.9 years for males; 25.5 years for females.

6 Sexuality

General Review Questions

1. What are the secondary sex characteristics for males and females?
2. List the phases of the human sexual response.
3. What are gender roles? How were your roles shaped by your parents, peers, schools, and the media?
4. What are "normal" sexual behaviors?
5. Identify the four major classes of sexual dysfunctions.

Practice Test #1

1. What is the correct sequence of the stages of sexual development?
   a. excitement, orgasm, plateau, resolution
   b. excitement, plateau, orgasm, resolution
   c. excitement, orgasm, resolution, plateau
   d. excitement, resolution, orgasm, plateau

2. What is the first sign of puberty in girls?
   a. widening of the hips
   b. development of pubic hair
   c. development of breast buds
   d. development of underarm hair

3. Which of the following defines androgyny?
   a. Androgyny is a combination of traditional masculine and feminine traits in a single person.
   b. Androgyny is the personal sense or awareness of being either masculine or feminine.
   c. Androgyny is the process by which a society transmits behavioral expectations to its individual members.
   d. Androgyny is the generalized way in which males and females express themselves the characteristics of each process.

4. What is the most common sexual desire disorder?
   a. dyspareunia
   b. premature ejaculation
   c. erectile dysfunction
   d. inhibited sexual desire

5. All of the following are part of the vulva, *except*
   a. labia minora.
   b. glans clitoris.
   c. vagina.
   d. mons veneris.

6. Ovulation usually occurs on the
   a. seventh day of the proliferatory phase.
   b. fourteenth day of the proliferatory phase.
   c. twenty-first day of the proliferatory phase.
   d. twenty-eighth day of the proliferatory phase.

7. Menopause results in
   a. increased production of testosterone.
   b. the presence of human chorionic gonadotropin.
   c. a sudden and permanent release of epinephrine.
   d. decreased estrogen levels.

8. Testes are responsible for the manufacture of
   a. progestin.
   b. follicle stimulating hormone.
   c. testosterone.
   d. androgens.

9. The structure where immature sperm ripen and reach full maturity is the
   a. testosterone.
   b. Cowper's gland.
   c. vasa deferentia.
   d. epididymis.

10. Emotional and sexual attraction to members of both sexes is called
    a. heterosexuality.
    b. homosexuality.
    c. bisexuality.
    d. androgyny.

11. During the human sexual response, vasocongestion occurs in the ________ phase.
    a. excitement/arousal
    b. plateau
    c. orgasm
    d. resolution

12. The avoidance or abstention from sexual activities with others is called
    a. celibacy.
    b. homosexuality.
    c. bisexuality.
    d. autosexuality.

13. A condition in which a person experiences sexual arousal by looking at or touching inanimate objects, such as underclothing or shoes, is called
    a. transvestitism.
    b. fetishism.
    c. voyeurism.
    d. sadomasochism.

14. The most frequent problem that causes people to seek out a sex therapist is
    a. erectile dysfunction.
    b. inhibited sexual desire.
    c. premature ejaculation.
    d. dyspareunia.

15. Ejaculation that occurs prior to or almost immediately following penile penetration of the vagina is called
    a. impotence.
    b. premature ejaculation.
    c. retarded ejaculation.
    d. erectile dysfunction.

Practice Test #2

1. Vaginismus and dyspareunia are common
    a. orgasm disorders.
    b. sexual pain disorders.
    c. sexual arousal disorders.
    d. sexual desire disorders.

2. Your personal sense of being masculine or feminine refers to your
    a. gender.
    b. gender role.
    c. gender identity.
    d. sexual acceptance.

3. The permanent cessation of menstruation is called
    a. amenhorrea.
    b. dysmenorrhea.
    c. menarche.
    d. menopause.

4. Sexual activity between an adult and a child is called
    a. pedophilia.
    b. fetishism.
    c. voyeurism.
    d. sadomasochism.

5. Sexual aversion disorder is a type of
    a. orgasm disorder.
    b. sexual pain disorder.
    c. sexual arousal disorder.
    d. sexual desire disorder.

6. The differential development of male and female gonads occurs at about the
    a. 8th week of fetal life.
    b. 20th week of fetal life.
    c. last trimester of fetal life.
    d. 2nd week after birth.

7. What is the hollow, muscular tube through which menstrual flow leaves the female's body called?
    a. fallopian tubes
    b. vagina
    c. uterus
    d. cervix

8. The lower end of the uterus that opens into the vagina is called the
    a. vagina.
    b. hymen.
    c. fallopian tubes.
    d. cervix.

9. What hormone signals the ovaries to begin producing estrogen?
    a. gonadotropin-releasing hormone
    b. follicle-stimulating hormone
    c. luteinizing hormone
    d. human chorionic gonadotropin

10. The internal male genitals include all of the following, *except*
    a. testes.
    b. scrotum.
    c. vasa deferentia.
    d. prostate.

11. The oral stimulation of a male's genitals is called
    a. cunnilingus.
    b. fellatio.
    c. coitus.
    d. autoerotic behaviors.

12. The exposure of one's genitals to strangers in public places is called
   a. pedophilia.
   b. exhibitionism.
   c. voyeurism.
   d. transsexualism.

13. Difficulty in achieving or maintaining a penile erection sufficient for intercourse is called
   a. erectile dysfunction.
   b. premature ejaculation.
   c. inhibited sexual desire.
   d. performance anxiety.

14. Sexual activities in which gratification is received by inflicting pain on a partner are called
   a. exhibitionism.
   b. fetishism.
   c. pedophilia.
   d. sadomasochism.

15. The most widely practiced form of sexual expression for most couples is
   a. cunnilingus.
   b. anal intercourse.
   c. vaginal intercourse.
   d. fellatio.

7 Reproductive Choices

General Review Questions

1. What conditions are necessary for conception?
2. Discuss the major purposes of prenatal care.
3. What are the signs of pregnancy?
4. How does the Norplant implant prevent pregnancy?
5. What risks are associated with abortion?

Practice Test #1

1. The fetus is especially subject to teratogens during the
   a. first trimester.
   b. second trimester.
   c. third trimester.
   d. fourth trimester.

2. The birth of the baby occurs during which stage of labor?
   a. first
   b. second
   c. third
   d. fourth

3. Which of the following birth alternatives allows the mother to deliver in a dark and quiet setting due to the belief that birth in a standard delivery room is traumatic?
   a. Lamaze method
   b. Harris method
   c. Bradley method
   d. Leboyer method

4. Five weeks after Barbara gave birth, she is still experiencing energy depletion, anxiety, mood swings, and depression. Barbara is suffering from
   a. postdelivery letdown.
   b. postlabor anxiety.
   c. postpartum depression.
   d. secondary pregnancy.

5. What is the most common method used for first-trimester abortions?
   a. dilation and evacuation
   b. vacuum aspiration
   c. dilation and curettage
   d. hysterotomy

6. Modern pregnancy tests are designed to detect the presence of
   a. HCG.
   b. LH.
   c. FSH.
   d. RU-486.

7. Toxic chemicals, pesticides, X-rays and other hazardous compounds that cause birth defects are referred to as
   a. carcinogens.
   b. teratogens.
   c. mutants.
   d. environmental assaults.

8. Detection of major health defects in a fetus as early as the fourteenth to eighteenth weeks of pregnancy can be determined by what procedure?
   a. ultrasound
   b. fetoscopy
   c. amniocentesis
   d. sonography

9. What happens during the second stage of labor?
   a. The amniotic sac breaks.
   b. The baby shifts into a head down position.
   c. The junction of the pubic bones loosens to permit expansion of the pelvic girth.
   d. The uterus works to push the baby through the birth canal.

10. What is the most popular birth alternative in the United States?
    a. Leboyer method
    b. Harris method
    c. Lamaze method
    d. Eclectic method

11. What occurs during the third stage of labor?
    a. Contractions become more rhythmic and painful.
    b. The amniotic sac breaks.
    c. The baby shifts into a head-down position.
    d. The placenta or afterbirth is expelled from the womb.

12. A soft, shallow cup made of thin latex rubber that is designed to cover the cervix and block access to the uterus is called a(n)
    a. condom.
    b. diaphragm.
    c. IUD.
    d. spermicidal sponge.

13. The type of contraceptive that consists of six silicon capsules that are surgically inserted under the skin of a woman's upper arm is called
    a. Depo-Provera.
    b. Norplant.
    c. progesterone inserts.
    d. intradermal devices.

14. What is the leading cause of infertility in women in the United States?
    a. pelvic inflammatory disease
    b. endometriosis
    c. low sperm count
    d. psychological stress

15. The fertilization of an egg in a test tube followed by transfer to a nutrient medium and subsequent transfer to the mother's body is called
    a. alternative insemination.
    b. in vitro fertilization.
    c. gamete intrafallopian transfer.
    d. nonsurgical embryo transfer.

Practice Test #2

1. Which of the following is a barrier method of contraception?
    a. condom
    b. oral contraceptives
    c. Norplant
    d. Depo-Provera

2. The cervical mucus method, the body temperature method, and the calendar method are all forms of
    a. barrier methods.
    b. hormonal methods.
    c. fertility awareness methods.
    d. surgical methods.

3. What prenatal test involves making a small incision in the abdominal and uterine walls and then inserting an optical viewer into the uterus to view the fetus directly?
    a. ultrasound
    b. fetoscopy
    c. amniocentesis
    d. chorionic villus sampling

4. The second stage of labor is called the
    a. transition stage.
    b. dilation stage.
    c. expulsion stage.
    d. afterbirth stage.

5. Janice chooses a birthing method that emphasizes no pain medication and little medical intervention in the birthing process. What birth alternative has she chosen?
    a. Bradley method
    b. Harris method
    c. Leboyer method
    d. Lamaze method

6. A collection of symptoms, including mental retardation, slowed nerve reflexes and small head size, that can appear in infants of women who drink too much alcohol during pregnancy is called
    a. teratogenic poisoning.
    b. fetal alcohol syndrome.
    c. Down syndrome.
    d. Tay-Sachs disease.

7. The most common birth defect found in babies born to older mothers is
    a. hemophilia.
    b. anencephaly.
    c. Down syndrome.
    d. sickle cell anemia.

8. The surgical procedure in which the female's fallopian tubes are closed or cut and cauterized to prevent access by sperm to released eggs is called
    a. tubal ligation.
    b. vasectomy.
    c. hysterectomy.
    d. abortion.

9. Medical care that is received prior to becoming pregnant and helps a woman assess her potential maternal health is called
   a. precoital care.
   b. preconception care.
   c. prenatal care.
   d. genetic counseling.

10. An ectopic pregnancy occurs when
   a. the fertilized egg implants outside the uterus.
   b. there is a chromosomal birth defect present.
   c. the mother is Rh positive and the fetus is Rh negative.
   d. the fetus is not viable.

11. Most oral contraceptives work through the
   a. use of synthetic follicle-stimulating hormones
   b. combined effects of synthetic estrogen and progesterone
   c. combined effects of synthetic testosterone and follicle-stimulating hormones
   d. use of estrogen-only hormones

12. Depo-Provera
   a. must be taken orally every 24 hours.
   b. consists of six silicone capsules that contain progesterone.
   c. is a long-acting synthetic progesterone that is injected intramuscularly every three months.
   d. must be inserted in the vagina at least 15 minutes prior to intercourse and left in place at least six hours afterwards.

13. A released ovum can survive for up to ___ hour(s) after ovulation, while sperm can live for as long as ___ day(s) in the vagina.
   a. 24 hours; 1 day
   b. 30 hours; 2 days
   c. 43 hours; 3 days
   d. 48 hours; 5 days

14. Sterilization of the male that consists of cutting and tying both vas deferens is called a
   a. vasectomy.
   b. tubal ligation.
   c. circumcision.
   d. None of the above

15. Low sperm count in males can result from
   a. the mumps virus.
   b. excessively tight underwear or outerwear.
   c. varicose veins.
   d. All of the above

8 Nutrition

General Review Questions

1. What factors influence when, what, and how much a person will eat?
2. List the six basic nutrients and the recommended U.S. dietary guidelines for each nutrient.
3. Describe the types of vegetarian diets.
4. What are the symptoms of food-borne illness?
5. List four steps students can take to maintain a nutritious diet within the confines of a restrictive budget.

Practice Test #1

1. Water is between __________ percent of total body weight.
   a. 20 and 30
   b. 30 and 40
   c. 40 and 50
   d. 50 and 60

2. What is the most common form of simple sugar in our diet?
   a. lactose
   b. sucrose
   c. fructose
   d. glucose

3. The two major forms of complex carbohydrates are
   a. starch and fruit.
   b. starch and fiber.
   c. fiber and fruit.
   d. fiber and lactose.

4. Which of the following nutrients helps move food through the digestive system?
   a. fat
   b. fiber
   c. starch
   d. minerals

5. Rick is a pesco-vegetarian. This means that he avoids
   a. flesh foods, but eats eggs.
   b. flesh foods, but eats dairy products.
   c. all foods of animal origin.
   d. meat but eat fish, dairy products, and eggs.

6. The Food Guide Pyramid recommends how many daily servings of fruit?
   a. 2-4
   b. 3-5
   c. 5-7
   d. 6-11

7. What is a common cause of anemia?
   a. ulcers
   b. cancers
   c. accidents
   d. iron deficiency

8. A toxic condiiton due to overuse of vitamin supplements is called
   a. microvitaminosis.
   b. megavitaminosis.
   c. hypovitaminosis.
   d. hypervitaminosis.

9. The feeling associated with physiological need to eat is called
   a. appetite.
   b. nutrition.
   c. hunger.
   d. nutritional survival.

10. The nutrient that aids in fluid and electrolyte balance, maintains pH balance, and transports molecules and cells throughout the body is
    a. water.
    b. minerals.
    c. vitamins.
    d. fat.

11. What type of carbohydrates are primarily found in grains, cereals, dark green leafy vegetables and cruciferous vegetables?
    a. simple carbohydrates
    b. complex carbohydrates
    c. glucose
    d. dextrose

12. The best way to increase dietary fiber in a diet is to
    a. eat more meat.
    b. eat more complex carbohydrates.
    c. decrease the amount of water to 3-4 glasses per day.
    d. decrease the amount of fruit while increasing beans and nuts.

13. Oat bran and dried beans are major sources of
    a. alpha cellulose.
    b. triglycerides.
    c. soluble fiber.
    d. insoluble fiber.

14. Compounds that facilitate the transportation of cholesterol in the blood to the liver for metabolism and elimination from the body are called
    a. plaque.
    b. high-density lipoproteins.
    c. low-density lipoproteins.
    d. very low-density lipoproteins.

15. The mineral folate has been shown to
    a. reduce the risk for colon cancer.
    b. decrease spina bifida and other neural tube defects in infants.
    c. decrease hypertension and diabetes.
    d. reduce the risk for breast cancer.

Practice Test #2

1. Fats that generally come from animals are called
    a. polyunsaturated fats.
    b. monounsaturated fats.
    c. saturated fats.
    d. low density lipoproteins.

2. What is the recommended number of servings each day from the bread, cereals, rice, and pasta group?
    a. 2-4 servings
    b. 3-5 servings
    c. 4-5 servings
    d. 6-11 servings

3. What organ determines which nutrients are stored, utilized, or excreted?
    a. pancreas
    b. liver
    c. stomach
    d. gall bladder

4. The entire digestive process takes
    a. 4 hours.
    b. 8 hours.
    c. 12 hours.
    d. 24 hours.

5. The second most common substance found in the body is
    a. fat.
    b. water.
    c. calcium.
    d. protein.

6. When too many calories are consumed, the
    a. excess is excreted from the body.
    b. body works harder to "burn" the calories.
    c. excess are converted into triglycerides in the liver, which are stored throughout our bodies.
    d. excess is circulated until it is burned as energy.

7. What nutrient supplies us with the energy needed to sustain normal daily activity?
    a. protein
    b. vitamins
    c. carbohydrates
    d. fiber

8. The process by which foods are broken down and either absorbed or excreted by the body is known as the
    a. digestive process.
    b. elimination process.
    c. metabolism process.
    d. nutritional process.

9. The majority of calories in the American diet come from
    a. proteins.
    b. carbohydrates.
    c. sugar.
    d. fat.

10. What nutrient is called the "body builder"?
   a. fats
   b. fiber
   c. proteins
   d. carbohydrates

11. Sodium, calcium, and chloride are examples of
   a. trace minerals.
   b. macrominerals.
   c. functional foods.
   d. proteins.

12. What is the most common nutrient deficiency worldwide?
   a. iron deficiency
   b. calcium deficiency
   c. chloride deficiency
   d. sodium deficiency

13. What type of simple sugar is found in corn syrup, honey, molasses, vegetables, and fruit?
   a. simple carbohydrates
   b. complex carbohydrates
   c. glucose
   d. dextrose

14. What is the most common form of fat circulating in the blood?
   a. cholesterol
   b. triglyceride
   c. saturated fat
   d. unsaturated fat

15. Which of the following is a water-soluble vitamin?
   a. Vitamin A
   b. Vitamin B
   c. Vitamin D
   d. Vitamin K

9 Managing Your Weight

General Review Questions

1. What factors are associated with the desire to be thin and attractive?
2. What factors affect basal metabolic rate?
3. What is social physique anxiety?
4. List the factors that determine the number of calories spent during physical activity.
5. What are three major eating disorders?

Practice Test #1

1. In general, a person is classified "obese" when they are
   a. 5%-10% above their ideal weight.
   b. 10%-20% above their ideal weight.
   c. 20%-30% above their ideal weight.
   d. 40%-50% above their ideal weight.

2. Sharon is 25% above her ideal weight. Traditionally, she would have been identified by nutritionists as
   a. mildly obese.
   b. moderately obese.
   c. severely obese.
   d. grossly overweight.

3. A body fat measurement technique that involves injecting radioactive substance into the body and allowing the substance to penetrate muscle tissue is called
   a. hydrostatic weighing.
   b. soft-tissue roentgenogram.
   c. bioelectrical impedance analysis.
   d. total body electrical conductivity.

4. The energy expenditure of the body under resting conditions at normal room temperature is called the
   a. basal metabolic rate (BMR).
   b. body mass index (BMI).
   c. bioelectrical impedance analysis (BIA).
   d. exercise metabolic rate (EMR).

5. Anorexia nervosa has been defined as a psychiatric disorder since
   a. 1678.
   b. 1873.
   c. 1921.
   d. 1978.

6. An accumulation of fat beyond what is considered normal for a person's age, sex, and body type is called
   a. body composition.
   b. obesity.
   c. overweight.
   d. body fat.

7. The ratio of lean body mass to fat body mass is
   a. obesity.
   b. body composition.
   c. overweight mass ratio.
   d. obesity ratio.

8. The technique of body fat assessment that utilizes electrical currents that are passed through fat and lean tissue is called
   a. body mass index.
   b. hydrostatic weight technique.
   c. bioelectrical impedance analysis.
   d. soft-tissue roentgenogram.

9. What is the ideal total body fat for women?
   a. 11-15%.
   b. 18-22%
   c. 23-29%
   d. 27-35%

10. What part of the brain regulates appetite and closely monitors levels of certain nutrients in the blood?
    a. pituitary gland
    b. hypothalamus
    c. cerebral cortex
    d. cerebellum

11. The theory of weight loss that proposes that a person's body has a set amount of weight at which it is programmed to be comfortable is called
    a. thermostatic maintenance theory.
    b. setpoint theory.
    c. plateau theory.
    d. endocrine balance theory.

12. What percentage of all the calories you consume on a given day go to support your basal metabolism (i.e. heartbeat, breathing, maintaining body temperature, etc.)?
    a. 20-30%
    b. 40-60%
    c. 60-70%
    d. 75-85%

13. An acute form of self-starvation motivated by a fear of gaining weight and a severe disturbance in the perception of one's body is called
    a. anorexia nervosa.
    b. bulimia.
    c. binge/purge syndrome.
    d. compulsive eating disorder.

14. A condition in which the body adapts to prolonged fasting or carbohydrate deprivation by converting body fat to ketones, which can be used as fuel for some brain activity is called
    a. caloric adaptation.
    b. carbohydrate synthesis.
    c. acidosis.
    d. ketones.

15. Fat necessary for normal physiological functioning is called
    a. body fat.
    b. essential fat.
    c. brown fat.
    d. storage fat.

Practice Test #2

1. One useful tool that has been in the news lately is a measure of regional fat distribution called the
   a. waist-to-height ratio.
   b. waist-to-arm ratio.
   c. waist-to-hip ratio.
   d. waist-to-chest ratio.

2. Studies of identical twins who were separated at birth and raised in different environments have provided evidence that obesity
   a. may be an inherited trait.
   b. has a metabolic explanation.
   c. is caused by a misfunctioning hyothalamus.
   d. is related to childhood eating habits.

3. A condition characterized by an excessive number of fat cells is called
   a. satiety.
   b. hypertrophy.
   c. hyperplasia.
   d. ketosis.

4. Which group of men are most likely to be overweight?
   a. men between ages 18 and 24
   b. men between ages 25 and 44
   c. men between ages 45 and 64
   d. men age 65 and older

5. What is the ideal total body fat for men?
   a. 5-10%
   b. 11-15%
   c. 16-20%
   d. 25-35%

6. What method of determining body fat measures the amount of water displaced when a person is completely submerged?
   a. skin-fold caliper test
   b. body mass index
   c. hydrostatic weighing technique
   d. bioelectrical impedance analysis

7. What medical standard is used to define obesity using an index of the relationship of height and weight?
   a. body composition index
   b. body mass index
   c. hydrostatic weight
   d. waist-to-hip ratio

8. What mechanism in the brain regulates metabolic activity according to caloric intake?
   a. adaptive thermogenesis
   b. hunger
   c. satiety
   d. appetite

9. The gland that is located in the throat that produces a hormone that regulates metabolism is the
   a. lymph gland.
   b. thyroid gland.
   c. adrenal gland.
   d. pancreas.

10. Eating food from fast-food restaurants is a problem because
   a. fast food is high in calories.
   b. fast food is eaten quickly so that there is not enough time for the "I'm full" signal.
   c. proportions tend to be bigger than they should be and tend to get eaten.
   d. All of the above

11. The desire to "look good" that has a destructive and sometimes disabling affect on one's ability to function effectively in relationships and interactions with others is called
   a. appearance anxiety.
   b. obesity anxiety.
   c. social physique anxiety.
   d. anorexia nervosa.

12. Approximately 90 percent of the daily calorie expenditures of most people occur as a result of
   a. basal metabolic rate.
   b. resting metabolic rate.
   c. exercise metabolic rate.
   d. sedentary metabolic rate.

13. The best way to improve one's chance for long-term success with weight loss is
   a. plan for nutrient-dense foods.
   b. plan for plateaus.
   c. chart your progress.
   d. All of the above

14. An eating disorder among clinically obese individuals who binge eat much more often than the typical obese person is called
   a. anorexia nervosa.
   b. bulimia nervosa.
   c. binge/purge syndrome.
   d. binge eating disorder.

15. A man would be considered obese if his body fat exceeds ___ percent of his total body mass while a woman is considered obese if her body fat is ___ percent of her total body mass.
   a. 15; 20
   b. 20; 30
   c. 35; 45
   d. 40; 50

10 Personal Fitness

General Review Questions

1. What is physical activity?
2. List the four components of physical fitness.
3. What is your target heart rate?
4. Why is flexibility important for fitness?
5. What first-aid treatment can be used for virtually all personal fitness injuries?

Practice Test #1

1. The treadmill running test is a type of
   a. graded exercise test.
   b. metabolic rate test.
   c. blood pressure test.
   d. duration test.

2. Keeping your heart beating at __________ of its maximum capability during exercise will result in the best cardiovascular fitness gains.
   a. 30 to 40%
   b. 50%
   c. 60%
   d. 70 to 90%

3. If you want to exercise at a conversational level, what should be your target heart rate?
   a. 40% of maximum
   b. 50% of maximum
   c. 70% of maximum
   d. 90% of maximum

4. Mary is 20 years old. What is her maximum heart rate?
   a. 70
   b. 135
   c. 195
   d. 200

5. The length of a daily physical activity of exercise period to improve aerobic capacity is
   a. no more than 10 minutes.
   b. 10-15 minutes.
   c. 15-20 minutes.
   d. 20-60 minutes.

6. A regular program of exercise designed to improve muscular strength and endurance in the major muscle groups is called a(n)
   a. flexibility training program.
   b. aerobic exercise program.
   c. repetition maximum program.
   d. resistance exercise program.

7. An Indian form of exercise widely practiced in the West today that promotes balance, coordination, flexibility and meditation is called
   a. body work.
   b. Tai chi.
   c. yoga.
   d. Zen.

8. The greatest amount of force in the muscles is produced during
   a. muscle overload.
   b. isometric muscle action.
   c. concentric muscle action.
   d. eccentric muscle action.

9. The primary category of physical activity known to improve cardiovascular fitness is
   a. aerobic exercise.
   b. anaerobic exercise.
   c. flexibility.
   d. body building.

10. The type of muscle action in which force is produced while the muscle shortens is called
    a. dynamic.
    b. static.
    c. concentric.
    d. eccentric.

11. The resistance provided by exercises that require your muscles to lift your body weight off the floor (i.e. situps, pushups, pullups) is called
    a. fixed resistance.
    b. variable resistance.
    c. accommodating resistance.
    d. body weight resistance.

12. The general term for any pain that occurs below the knee and above the ankle is
    a. shin splints.
    b. tendinitis.
    c. muscle cramps.
    d. muscle strain.

13. Superior stretching techniques that are best performed with a certified athletic trainer or physical therapist are called
    a. static stretching techniques.
    b. proprioceptive neuromuscular facilitation.
    c. ballistic stretching techniques.
    d. tandem stretching techniques.

14. The amount of force a muscle is capable of exerting is called
    a. muscular efficiency.
    b. muscular strength.
    c. muscular endurance.
    d. muscular overload.

15. A condition in which the body's rate of heat production exceeds its ability to cool itself is known as
    a. hypothermia.
    b. heat stress.
    c. compression.
    d. muscle strain.

Practice Test #2

1. After you run on a treadmill for 45 minutes, you should have a cool-down period to allow
   a. your stomach muscles to relax.
   b. lactic acid and carbon dioxide to be removed more rapidly from the blood.
   c. your blood pressure to return to normal.
   d. None of the above

2. Which principle refers to the way in which a specific body system responds to the physiological demands placed on it?
   a. tension principle
   b. overload principle
   c. specificity of training principle
   d. setpoint principle

3. When Joe was playing baseball, he broke an arm when he slid into homeplate. What type of injury is this called?
   a. underuse injury
   b. overuse injury
   c. traumatic injury
   d. intensity injury

4. What is RICE?
   a. components of the setpoint theory
   b. components of first-aid treatment
   c. components of exercise
   d. components of cross-training

5. What is known as the conversational level of exericse?
   a. target heart rate of 30 percent of maximum
   b. target heart rate of 50 percent of maximum
   c. target heart rate of 70 percent of maximum
   d. target heart rate of 90 percent of maximum

6. People who exercise regularly often report
   a. an increased ability to cope with stress.
   b. an increased self-esteem.
   c. feeling good about personal appearance.
   d, All of the above

7. Muscle endurance is
   a. the force exerted by a muscle that is less than or equal to the resistance.
   b. a muscle's ability to exert force repeatedly without fatiguing.
   c. the length of time a particular movement can be sustained by a muscle or muscle group.
   d. a withering of muscle tissue that can result from injury or disease.

8. The systematic performance of exercise at a specified frequency, intensity, and duration to achieve a desired level of physical fitness is called
   a. fitness training.
   b. physical fitness.
   c. exercise training.
   d. physical endurance.

9. The recommended minimum number of times per week that a physical activity and/or exercise should be done to reach aerobic fitness is
   a. 1 time per week.
   b. 3 times per week.
   c. 5 times per week.
   d. 7 times per week.

10. Increased levels of high density lipoproteins can diminish the risk of
    a. diabetes.
    b. osteoarthritis.
    c. osteoporosis.
    d. cardiovascular disease.

11. The type of resistance that provides a "constant load" on the muscle throughout the entire range of motion is called
    a. body weight resistance.
    b. static resistance.
    c. fixed resistance.
    d. accommodating resistance.

12. The use of resistance that is altered throughout the range of motion so that the effort by the muscle is more consistent throughout the full range of motion is called
    a. static resistance.
    b. muscular function resistance.
    c. variable resistance.
    d. isometric resistance.

13. The maximal volume of oxygen consumed by muscles during exercise is
    a. flexibility.
    b. muscle endurance.
    c. aerobic capacity.
    d. maximum oxygen capacity.

14. Injuries that result from the cumulative effects of day-after-day stress placed on tendons, muscles, and joints are called
    a. overuse injuries.
    b. traumatic injuries.
    c. overtraining injuries.
    d. repetitive injuries.

15. Techniques to gradually lengthen a muscle to an elongated position (to the point of discomfort) and hold that position for 10 to 30 seconds is called
    a. dynamic stretching.
    b. static stretching.
    c. variable stretching.
    d. concentric stretching.

11 Addictions and Addictive Behavior

General Review Questions

1. What are the criteria for diagnosis of an addiction?
2. What are the signs of addiction?
3. Describe the cycle of psychological addiction.
4. What are the components of an effective intervention?
5. The most effective treatment for addiction is based on what model?

Practice Test #1

1. Academic failure is an example of which addictive symptom?
   a. denial
   b. loss of control
   c. obsession and compulsion
   d. negative consequences

2. Melissa's food addiction began when she repeatedly sought the illusion of relief through food to avoid her feelings of rejection by her stepfather. This pattern is called
   a. acting out.
   b. nurturing through avoidance.
   c. addictive logic.
   d. addictive reaction.

3. Jack is addicted to the Internet. He is so preoccupied with talking in chat rooms that he skips classes to get online. His preoccupation with the Internet characterizes what symptom of addiction?
   a. denial
   b. obsession and compulsion
   c. loss of control
   d. negative consequences

4. What is the first step in the cycle of psychological addiction?
   a. emotional pain
   b. craving for relief
   c. short-term pain relief
   d. depression or guilt or shame

5. Ben used to get "high" after drinking a six-pack of beer. But over time, he finds that he needs to drink a 12-pack to get the same effects. This relates to
   a. withdrawal.
   b. tolerance.
   c. relapse.
   d. detoxification.

6. Habits differ from addictions in that
   a. habits can be broken without too much discomfort.
   b. the repetition of the behavior occurs by compulsion and considerable comfort is experienced if the behavior is not performed.
   c. they result in such negative consequences as physical damage, financial problems, and/or family dissolution.
   d. they are self-destructive.

7. Michael is in a fraternity and drinks heavily at social events or other functions. He does not believe that his drinking pattern is a problem, even though his grades have suffered as a result of his drinking. He is experiencing
   a. a habit.
   b. an obsession.
   c. a compulsion.
   d. denial.

8. Biochemical messengers that exert influence at specific receptor site(s) on the nerve cells are called
   a. neurons.
   b. hormones.
   c. neurotransmitters.
   d. euphoric cells.

9. The phenomenon in which progressively larger doses of a drug are needed to produce the desired effects is called
   a. tolerance.
   b. withdrawal.
   c. dependency.
   d. addiction.

10. Common addictions that are mood-altering are called
    a. process addictions.
    b. obsessions.
    c. compulsion addictions.
    d. interdependence.

11. The major life event that is the most common trigger for excessive drinking among the elderly is
    a. a second marriage.
    b. divorce.
    c. retirement.
    d. death of a spouse.

12. The model of addiction that proposes that people learn behaviors by watching parents, caregivers, and significant others is known as
    a. societal influences model.
    b. stimulus-response model.
    c. social learning theory.
    d. behavioral intent model.

13. The relationship pattern in which a person is thought to be "addicted to the addict" is known as
    a. enabling.
    b. codependent.
    c. post-traumatic stress.
    d. control-controller relationship.

14. The early abstinence period during which an addict adjust physically and cognitively to being free from the influences of the addiction refers to
    a. denial.
    b. abstinence.
    c. detoxification.
    d. interdependence.

15. An isolated occurrence of or full return to addictive behaviors is called
    a. response mechanism.
    b. relapse.
    c. withdrawal.
    d. recovery.

Practice Test #2

1. What sign of addiction refers to the inability to reliably predict whether any isolated occurrence of the behavior will be healthy or damaging?
    a. denial
    b. loss of control
    c. negative consequences
    d. obsession and compulsion

2. Who of the following are at risk for developing a gambling addiction?
    a. women
    b. higher-income individuals
    c. whites
    d. divorced individuals

3. Treatment and recovery for any addiction generally begins with
    a. abstinence.
    b. intervention.
    c. nurturing through avoidance.
    d. relapse.

4. Which of the following was *not* a criterion for the traditional diagnosis of an addiction?
    a. abstinence syndrome
    b. denial
    c. relapse
    d. an associated pattern of pathological behavior

5. Sex addicts confuse
    a. physical attraction with mental attraction.
    b. love with lust.
    c. nature with nurture.
    d. intensity of sexual arousal with intimacy.

6. What is the primary outcome of dysfunctional relationships?
    a. trauma
    b. divorce
    c. codependence
    d. co-addictiveness

7. What teaches people how to recognize the signs of imminent relapse and develop a predetermined plan for responding to these signs?
    a. sobriety
    b. addictive cycle
    c. detoxification
    d. relapse prevention

8. A series of temporary physical and psychological symptoms that occur when the addict stops the addictive behavior is known as
   a. physiological dependence.
   b. withdrawal.
   c. tolerance.
   d. addiction.

9. To be addictive, a behavior must
   a. have the potential to produce a positive mood change.
   b. produce a positively reinforcing response.
   c. result in a physiological dependency.
   d. be reinforced by a set of events that support the addiction.

10. What is the severest side effect of withdrawal?
   a. depression
   b. delirium tremens
   c. irritability
   d. convulsions

11. The theory that proposes that addiction is caused by a variety of factors operating together is known as the
   a. sociocultural influences theory.
   b. social learning theory.
   c. life events model.
   d. biopsychosocial model.

12. People who knowingly or unknowingly protect addicts from the natural consequences of their behavior are
   a. codependents.
   b. enablers.
   c. coaddicts.
   d. rescuers.

13. A planned process of confrontation by significant others including spouse, parents, children, boss, and friends is called
   a. an intervention.
   b. denial.
   c. the treatment process.
   d. enabling.

14. People who work out compulsively to try to meet needs of nurturance, intimacy, self-esteem, and self-competency have a(n)
   a. money addiction.
   b. work addiction.
   c. exercise addiction.
   d. shopping addiction.

15. Codependents have difficulty
   a. experiencing appropriate levels of self-esteem.
   b. setting healthy boundaries.
   c. taking care of their own adult needs and desires.
   d. All of the above

12 Drinking Responsibly

General Review Questions

1. What are the factors that influence how quickly alcohol is absorbed by the body?
2. How does alcohol affect the immune system?
3. What are the unique problems of adult children of alcoholics?
4. What are the annual costs of alcohol abuse to society?
5. When does an alcoholic seek help?

Practice Test #1

1. As Ted was growing up, his function in the family was to have the focus on him, taking the heat off of everyone else. What was his role?
   a. mascot
   b. family hero
   c. scapegoat
   d. lost child

2. A man and a woman weigh the same and drink the same amount of alcohol over the same amount of time. Whose blood alcohol content will be higher?
   a. They will be the same.
   b. The man's will be 10% higher.
   c. The man's will be 30% higher.
   d. The woman's will be 30% higher.

3. An effective method of helping an alcoholic to confront the disease is through a process called
   a. intervention.
   b. confrontation.
   c. intermediary assistance.
   d. reality orientation.

4. Withdrawal takes from
   a. 24 to 72 hours.
   b. 1 to 3 weeks.
   c. 4 to 6 weeks.
   d. 3 to 6 months.

5. Research has shown that less than 1% percent of recovered alcoholics are able to resume drinking on a limited social basis.
   a. 1
   b. 10
   c. 25
   d. 50

6. The majority of alcohol is absorbed into the bloodstream in the
   a. mouth.
   b. stomach.
   c. small intestine.
   d. large intestine.

7. Approximately 84 percent of students consume alcoholic beverages.
   a. 20
   b. 43
   c. 65
   d. 84

8. Lindsay has joined a sorority, and when she goes to a social with a fraternity she usually has five or six drinks in a row. This type of high risk drinking is called
   a. alcohol overconsumption.
   b. binge drinking.
   c. drinking overabuse.
   d. alcoholic addiction.

9. The alcohol content in beer is usually
   a. 2-6 percent.
   b. 6-10 percent.
   c. 12-15 percent.
   d. 15-19 percent.

10. Doug likes to have a drink to help him feel slightly relaxed. The blood alcohol concentration level that produces this effect is
    a. .02.
    b. .05.
    c. .08.
    d. .10.

11. At a party, Roger has been "shooting" tequila in large amounts over a short time. He has become unconscious and cannot be aroused. In addition, his breathing is irregular and his skin is bluish. Unless he gets immediate help, he can die from
    a. alcohol abuse.
    b. pancreatitis.
    c. alcohol poisoning.
    d. delirium tremors.

12. Liver deterioration caused by fibrous scar tissue is called
    a. cardiomyopathy.
    b. antithrombotic disease.
    c. liver hepatitis.
    d. liver fibrosis.

13. When a mother consumes alcohol during pregnancy, which of the following disorders can result?
    a. sudden infant death syndrome
    b. pancreatitis
    c. fetal alcohol syndrome
    d. osteoporosis

14. The primary action of ethanol within the central nervous system is to
    a. reduce the frequency of nerve transmissions and impulses at the synaptic junctions.
    b. increase the frequency of nerve transmissions and impulses at the synaptic junctions.
    c. reduce the frequency of nerve transmissions and increase the impulses at the synaptic junctions.
    d. increase the frequency of nerve transmissions and decrease the impulses at the synaptic junctions.

15. Ed is an alcoholic who grew up in a family with an alcoholic father. Alcohol was an accepted practice by his parents and grandparents. In fact, his father took him out drinking to celebrate his 21st birthday. Ed is a
    a. Type I alcoholic.
    b. Type II alcoholic.
    c. Type III alcoholic.
    d. Type II reactive alcoholic.

Practice Test #2

1. Sue grew up in a dysfunctional family. She always provided comic relief and was the "fun" one in the family who offset her father's alcoholism. What was Sue's role?
    a. mascot
    b. lost child
    c. family hero
    d. scapegoat

2. What is the most common preventable cause of mental impairments in the Western world?
    a. Down syndrome
    b. cerebral palsy
    c. fetal alcohol syndrome
    d. Tay-Sachs disease

3. The process by which addicts end their dependence on a drug and which is commonly carried out in a medical facility is called
    a. recovery.
    b. intervention.
    c. detoxification.
    d. aversion therapy.

4. Alcohol is metabolized in the
    a. stomach.
    b. liver.
    c. lower third of the small intestine.
    d. upper third of the small intestine.

5. The process whereby yeast organisms break down plant sugars to yield ethanol and carbon dioxide is called
    a. fermentation.
    b. distillation.
    c. mashation.
    d. alcoholization.

6. Blood alcohol concentration (BAC) is the
    a. concentration of plant sugars in the blood stream.
    b. percentage of alcohol in a beverage.
    c. level of alcohol content in the blood before becoming drunk.
    d. ratio of alcohol to the total blood volume.

7. Among women, moderate levels of alcohol consumption has been linked with
    a. vaginal cancer.
    b. ovarian cancer.
    c. uterine cancer.
    d. breast cancer.

8. A child in a dysfunctional family becomes passive and quietly withdraws when his parents fight over how much his father has been drinking. What role has the child adopted?
    a. scapegoat
    b. family hero
    c. mascot
    d. lost child

9. If whisky is 80 proof, what is the percentage of alcohol in the drink?
   a. 20%
   b. 40%s
   c. 60%
   d. 80%

10. A driver's BAC depends on
    a. his or her weight and body fat.
    b. the water content in his or her body tissue.
    c. the volume of the alcohol.
    d. All of the above

11. People who drink moderately experience which of the following effects?
    a. shrinkage in brain size
    b. shrinkage in brain weight
    c. a loss in some degree of intellectual ability
    d. All of the above

12. A syndrome describing children with a history of prenatal alcohol exposure but without all of the physical or behavioral symptoms of FAS is called
    a. alcoholic behavioral syndrome.
    b. fetal alcoholic hepatitis.
    c. fetal alcohol effects.
    d. fetal alcoholic abuse.

13. Which of the following characterizes Type 2 alcoholics?'
    a. seek social approval
    b. lack inhibition
    c. avoid harmful situations
    d. concerned about the thoughts and feelings of others

14. What percent of traffic fatalities are alcohol-related?
    a. 16%
    b. 25%
    c. 38%
    d. 55%

15. Two distinct subtypes of alcoholism support what causal factor in alcoholism?
    a. social
    b. cultural
    c. biological
    d. learned

13 Tobacco and Caffeine

General Review Questions

1. List the dangerous chemicals in tobacco smoke.
2. What are the physical effects of nicotine?
3. Describe the warning signs of oral cancer.
4. Describe the most common therapy techniques for quitting smoking.
5. What health problems are associated with long-term caffeine use?

Practice Test #1

1. What is the single most preventable cause of death in the United States?
   a. alcohol use
   b. illegal drug use
   c. tobacco use
   d. prescription drug abuse

2. Of all the deaths in the United States, how many are related to tobacco?
   a. one of every two deaths
   b. one of every three deaths
   c. one of every five deaths
   d. one of every ten deaths

3. Between 1990 and 1999, cigarette smoking among U.S. college students
   a. decreased 32 percent.
   b. decreased 3 percent.
   c. increased 3 percent.
   d. increased 32 percent.

4. Which age group is the new target for tobacco advertisers?
   a. 12-17 year olds
   b. 18-24 year olds
   c. 24-44 year olds
   d. 45-64 year olds

5. Smoking can cause emphysema, a chronic disease which affects the
   a. salivary glands.
   b. esophagus.
   c. larynx.
   d. lungs.

6. What type of tobacco comes in the form of loose leaf, plug, or twist?
   a. snuff
   b. chewing tobacco
   c. cigarettes
   d. cigars

7. While smoking her first cigarette, Nancy begins to get dizzy, lightheaded, nauseated, and clammy skin. Most likely Nancy is experiencing
   a. nicotine poisoning.
   b. nicotine withdrawal.
   c. nicotine intolerance.
   d. nicotine overdose.

8. Nicotine acts as a(n) _________ on the central nervous system.
   a. stimulant
   b. analgesic
   c. depressant
   d. hallucinogenic

9. Smokers have a __________ percent higher death rate from heart disease than do nonsmokers.
   a. 25
   b. 36
   c. 47
   d. 70

10. A chronic disease in which the alveoli are destroyed, making breathing difficult is
    a. chronic obstructive lung disorder.
    b. stroke.
    c. emphysema.
    d. sudden infant death syndrome.

11. The cigarette, pipe, or cigar smoke breathed by nonsmokers is called
    a. secondhand smoke.
    b. sidestream smoke.
    c. nicotine poisoning.
    d. nicotine intolerance.

12. Which of the following is *not* a symptom of nicotine withdrawal?
    a. nausea
    b. vomiting
    c. headaches
    d. hypertension

symptoms

13. How many years must an ex-smoker be smoke-free to expect to live out his/her normal life span?
    a. 2 years
    b. 5 years
    c. 10 years
    d. 15 years

14. A condition characterized by leathery white patches inside the mouth produced by contact with the irritants in tobacco juice is known as
    a. leukoplakia.
    b. neoplasm.
    c. dental fissures.
    d. oral cancer.

15. A derivative of the chemical family of stimulants called xanthines is found in
    a. snuff.
    b. nicotine.
    c. tobacco.
    d. coffee.

Practice Test #2

1. A type of antismoking therapy where the act of smoking is paired with some sort of noxious stimulus so that smoking itself is perceived as unpleasant is called
    a. aversion therapy.
    b. operant conditioning.
    c. self-control.
    d. nicotine withdrawal.

2. In developing countries promotional cigarette ads are often aimed at
women because
    a. half of the men already smoke but few women do.
    b. men in developing countries are not swayed by advertising.
    c. laws prohibit misleading advertising aimed at men.
    d. women control the purchasing decisions.

3. Long-term caffeine use has been linked to all of the following
serious health problems, *except*
    a. heart disease.
    b. cancer.
    c. mental dysfunction.
    d. high blood pressure.

4. Most smoking-related deaths in the United States result from
    a. coronary heart disease and stroke.
    b. coronary heart disease and chronic lung disease.
    c. stroke and lung cancer.
    d. lung cancer and coronary heart disease.

5. The thick brownish substance condensed from particulate matter .in cigarette smoke is called
    a. tar.
    b. nicotine.
    c. chewing tobacco.
    d. carbon monoxide.

6. Which of the following is *not* a physical effect of nicotine stimulation?
    a. constriction of blood vessels
    b. decrease in stomach contractions
    c. increase sensation in the taste buds
    d. increased blood pressure

7. What is the leading cause of cancer death from smoking?
    a. throat cancer
    b. colon cancer
    c. lung cancer
    d. stomach cancer

8. Stickiness of red blood cells associated with blood clots is called
    a. clumping.
    b. platelet adhesiveness.
    c. elevated HDLs.
    d. stroke.

9. Daily smoking of one cigar
    a. is a safe practice that does not increase a person's risk for health problems.
    b. increases a person's risk for cancer of the lip, tongue, mouth, larynx and lungs.
    c. is safe for others who may be exposed to the smoke.
    d. is safe because cigars do not have the harmful ingredients contained in cigarettes.

10. Babies born to women who smoke during pregnancy are more likely to die from
    a. congenital heart failure.
    b. pneumonia.
    c. sudden infant death syndrome.
    d. infantile paralysis.

11. Smoking has been shown to affect women by
    a. causing women to begin menopause one to two years earlier.
    b. contributing to the development of osteoporosis.
    c. increasing the risk of death from emphysema or chronic bronchitis.
    d. All of the above

12. What age group has the highest percentage of smokers?
    a. 15-24 year olds
    b. 25-44 year olds
    c. 44-55 year olds
    d. 55 year olds and older

13. The financial costs for smoking in the workplace include all of the following, *except*
    a. absenteeism.
    b. loss of productivity.
    c. training to replace employees who die prematurely.
    d. loss of time due to excessive breaks.

14. Caffeine acts as a(n) stimulant on the central nervous system.
    a. stimulant
    b. analgesic
    c. depressant
    d. hallucinogenic

15. Sensory disturbance from caffeine may be experienced after 10 cups of coffee within a 24-hour period.
    a. 3
    b. 5
    c. 7
    d. 10

14 Illicit Drugs

General Review Questions

1. What are the six categories of drugs?
2. What are the health problems found in cocaine-affected babies?
3. List the physiological effects of LSD.
4. Who are the primary users of anabolic steroids?
5. What is the best approach to drug education?

Practice Test #1

1. The most frequently used route of administration of drugs is
   a. inhalation.
   b. oral ingestion.
   c. intravenous injection.
   d. subcutaneous injection.

2. Drugs with the highest potential for abuse are included in
   a. Schedule I.
   b. Schedule II.
   c. Schedule IV.
   d. Schedule V.

3. Marijuana has medicinal value, including treatment for
   a. heart disease and brain cancer.
   b. cataracts and lung cancer.
   c. chemotherapy and glaucoma.
   d. depression and heart disease.

4. What route of administration does insulin replacement therapy take?
   a. inunction
   b. oral ingestion
   c. subcutaneous injection
   d. intramuscular injection

5. Applying patches to the skin behind your ear to prevent motion sickness is an example of a(n)
   a. inunction.
   b. inhalation.
   c. injection.
   d. suppository.

6. A powerful stimulant drug made from the leaves of the South American coca shrub is called
   a. LSD.
   b. cocaine.
   c. marijuana.
   d. amphetamines.

7. The most powerful distillate of cocaine is
   a. powdered cocaine.
   b. freebase cocaine.
   c. crack.
   d. rock cocaine.

8. What is the active ingredient in marijuana?
   a. PCP
   b. MDMA
   c. LSD
   d. THC

9. A dark, brown sticky substance made from morphine is
   a. codeine.
   b. black tar heroin.
   c. morphine.
   d. opium.

10. A synthetic opiod that is used in the treatment of people addicted to heroin is called
    a. codeine.
    b. morphine.
    c. methadone.
    d. methamphetamine.

11. An image (auditory or visual) that is perceived but is not real is called a
    a. blackout.
    b. flashback.
    c. synesthesia.
    d. hallucination.

12. Ecstasy is categorized as a
    a. narcotic.
    b. depressant.
    c. hallucinogenic.
    d. designer drug.

13. Rubber cement, model glue, spot removers, and gasoline are examples of
    a. depressants.
    b. inhalants.
    c. stimulants.
    d. psychedelics.

14. Artificial forms of the hormone testosterone that promote muscle growth and strength are called
   a. aerobic steriods.
   b. anabolic steriods.
   c. anaerobic steroids.
   d. erogenic drugs.

15. Which of the following is *not* a narcotic?
   a. morphine
   b. methamphetamine
   c. codeine
   d. heroin

Practice Test #2

1. Applying a small adhesive patch to introdcue a prescription medicaiton into the body through the skin is called
   a. inhalation.
   b. inunction.
   c. subcutaneous injection.
   d. oral administration.

2. What is the most frequently used illicit drug?
   a. PCP
   b. marijuana
   c. crack
   d. heroin

3. Which of the following is *not* an opiate?
   a. heroin
   b. codeine
   c. morphine
   d. hashish

4. Over-the-counter preparations are included under which drug schedule?
   a. Schedule I
   b. Schedule II
   c. Schedule IV
   d. Schedule V

5. Heroin is included under what drug schedule?
   a. Schedule I
   b. Schedule II
   c. Schedule IV
   d. Schedule V

6. Drugs with a high potential for abuse and addiction and have no medical use are categorized as
   a. Schedule I drugs.
   b. Schedule II drugs.
   c. Schedule III drugs.
   d. Schedule IV drugs.

7. A derivative of opium that is sometimes used to relieve pain is
   a. morphine.
   b. heroin.
   c. codeine.
   d. methadone.

8. The narcotic used in cough syrups and certain painkillers is
   a. morphine.
   b. cocaine.
   c. codeine.
   d. heroin.

9. The most common route of administration for heroin addicts is
   a. inhalation.
   b. intravenous injection.
   c. ingestion.
   d. inunction.

10. According to the "schedule" of drugs, cocaine is categorized as a
   a. Schedule I drug.
   b. Schedule II drug.
   c. Schedule III drug.
   d. Schedule IV drug.

11. Opiate-like hormones that are manufactured in the human brain and contribute to feelings of well-being are
   a. endorphins.
   b. acetaminaphine.
   c. adrenaline.
   d. acetylcholine.

12. The group of drugs whose primary pharmacological effect is characterized by confusion and disorientation in the user is called
   a. narcotics.
   b. deliriants.
   c. stimulants.
   d. depressants.

13. A hallucinogenic drug derived from the peyote cactus is called
    a. mescaline.
    b. methamphetamine.
    c. LSD.
    d. psilocybin.

14. Which of the following is a deliriant?
    a. Tetrahydrocannabinol (THC)
    b. Phencyclidine (PCP)
    c. Ecstasy (MDMA)
    d. Lysergic Acid Diethylamide (LSD)

15. LSD is a(n)
    a. opiate.
    b. deliriant.
    c. stimulant.
    d. psychedelic.

15 Cardiovascular Disease

General Review Questions

1. List the risk factors for cardiovascular disease.
2. What are the risk factors for cardiovascular disease that we cannot prevent or control?
3. Discuss the common treatments for angina pectoris.
4. List the specific factors that cause secondary hypertension?
5. What are the reasons for the widespread neglect of the signs of heart disease in women?

Practice Test #1

1. Small blood vessels that permit the exchange of oxygen, carbon dioxide, nutrients, and waste products with body cells are called
   a. arterioles.
   b. valves.
   c. capillaries.
   d. venules.

2. Brett is at the cardiac center having tests for an abnormally slow heartbeat. His condition is called
   a. thrombosis.
   b. tachycardia.
   c. bradycardia.
   d. fibrillation.

3. What serves as a form of natural pacemaker for the heart?
   a. aortic valve
   b. pulmonary valve
   c. tricuspid valve
   d. sinoatrial node

4. Of all the major types of CVD, what is the single greatest killer?
   a. stroke
   b. atherosclerosis
   c. coronary heart disease
   d. congenital heart disease

5. Calcium channel blockers and beta blockers are two major types of drugs used to treat
   a. angina pectoris.
   b. coronary heart disease.
   c. arrhythmia.
   d. atherosclerosis.

6. Joanne drinks an excessive amount of caffeine and smokes a pack of cigarettes a day, which contributed to experiencing an irregularity in heartbeat, known as
   a. angina pectoris.
   b. arrhythmia.
   c. rheumatic heart disease.
   d. atherosclerosis.

7. What is the leading cause of death in the United States?
   a. strokes
   b. traffic fatalities
   c. cardiovascular diseases
   d. cancer

8. What part of the cardiovascular system carries blood away from the heart?
   a. atrium
   b. veins
   c. capillaries
   d. arteries

9. A blockage of the normal blood supply to an area of the heart is called
   a. a stroke.
   b. a coronary thrombosis.
   c. a heart attack.
   d. angina pectoris.

10. An irregular heartbeat is called
   a. fibrillation.
   b. bradycardia.
   c. tachycardia.
   d. arrhythmia.

11. What drug is used to dilate veins and reduce the amount of blood returning to the heart and thus lessen its workload?
   a. Nitroglycerin
   b. Inderal
   c. Prinivil
   d. Lopressor

12. When the blood supply to the brain is cut off, the result may be a(n)
   a. myocardial infarction.
   b. thrombosis.
   c. stroke.
   d. aneurysm.

13. An abnormally fast heartbeat is known as
   a. arrhythmia.
   b. tachycardia.
   c. vasodilation.
   d. bradycardia.

14. The diagnostic technique that uses powerful magnets to look inside the body is called
   a. radionuclide imaging.
   b. magnetic resonance imaging.
   c. digital cardiac angiography.
   d. cardiomagnetic angioplasty.

15. A surgical technique whereby a blood vessel is implanted to bypass a blocked artery is called
   a. angioplasty.
   b. electrocardiogram.
   c. pacemaker implantation.
   d. coronary bypass surgery.

Practice Test #2

1. The heart is a __________-chambered pump.
   a. two
   b. three
   c. four
   d. five

2. The development of new, small blood vessels that reroute needed blood through other areas as a result of minor heart blockage is called
   a. coronary circulation.
   b. collateral circulation.
   c. converse circulation.
   d. coronary thrombosis.

3. Which of the following is *not* a cause of stroke?
   a. angina
   b. thrombus
   c. embolus
   d. aneurysm

4. What type of cardiovascular disease is an inflammatory disease?
   a. stroke
   b. arrhythmia
   c. atherosclerosis
   d. coronary heart disease

5. The two upper chambers of the heart are called
   a. atria.
   b. arteries.
   c. veins.
   d. ventricles.

6. Severe chest pain occurring as a result of reduced oxygen flow to the heart is called
   a. angina pectoris.
   b. arrhythmias.
   c. myocardial infarction.
   d. congestive heart failure.

7. What type of heart disease is caused by untreated streptococcal infection of the throat?
   a. congestive heart failure
   b. congenital heart disease
   c. rheumatic heart disease
   d. coronary thrombosis

8. What is the greatest alterable risk factor for CVD?
   a. smoking
   b. diet
   c. exercise
   d. hypertension

9. The blood pressure value that refers to the pressure being applied to the walls of the arteries when the heart contracts is
   a. diastolic pressure.
   b. systolic pressure.
   c. normal pressure.
   d. contraction pressure.

10. The diagnostic technique in which a needle-thin catheter is threaded through blocked arteries of the heart, a dye injected, and an X-ray is taken to find the blocked areas is called
   a. angiography.
   b. angioplasty.
   c. electrocardiogram.
   d. positron emission tomography.

11. Under normal circumstances, the body contains __________ quarts of blood.
   a. 4
   b. 6
   c. 8
   d. 10

12. A general term for the thickening or hardening of the arteries is
   a. myocardial infarction.
   b. cerebrovascular accident.
   c. atherosclerosis.
   d. arrhythmia.

13. A weakening in a blood vessel that causes it to bulge and, in severe cases, burst is called
   a. congestive heart failure.
   b. angina pectoris.
   c. an aneurysm.
   d. an arrhythmia.

14. Reperfusion therapy for a heart attack is called
   a. nitroglycerin.
   b. thrombolysis.
   c. angioplasty.
   d. angiogram.

15. The average adult heart at rest beats ________ times per minute.
   a. 45 to 55
   b. 50 to 60
   c. 60 to 70
   d. 70 to 80

16 Cancer

General Review Questions

1. What are the four classifications of cancer?
2. List the symptoms of lung cancer.
3. What is the ABCD rule for malignant melanoma?
4. List the high-tech diagnostic techniques that are used to detect cancer.
5. Describe the preventive actions an individual can take to prevent cancer.

Practice Test #1

1. Breast cancer is an example of a
   a. lymphoma.
   b. sarcoma.
   c. carcinoma.
   d. leukemia.

2. What involves removal of the breast, lymph nodes, pectoral muscles, all fat, and underlying tissue?
   a. lumpectomy
   b. simple mastectomy
   c. modified readical mastectomy
   d. radical mastectomy

3. What is the most common carcinogen?
   a. asbestos
   b. pesticides
   c. smog
   d. tar in cigarettes

4. What are the most common sites for cancers?
   a. epithelial tissues
   b. mesodermal tissues
   c. blood-forming parts of the body
   d. lymphatic system

5. Tamoxifen is often an alternative to chemotherapy for many women with
   a. lung cancer.
   b. breast cancer.
   c. ovarian cancer.
   d. cervical cancer.

6. Human papilloma virus has been linked to
   a. testicular cancer.
   b. breast cancer.
   c. cervical cancer.
   d. ovarian cancer.

7. Cancer of the blood-forming parts of the body, particularly the bone marrow and spleen, is called
   a. lymphoma.
   b. leukemia.
   c. carcinoma.
   d. sarcoma.

8. The second leading cause of cancer death in males is
   a. lung cancer.
   b. breast cancer.
   c. testicular cancer.
   d. prostate cancer.

9. The treatment of skin cancer that involves tissue destruction by freezing is called
   a. surgery.
   b. cryosurgery.
   c. electrodesication.
   d. radiation therapy.

10. Cancers that occur in the mesodermal layers of tissue (i.e., bones, muscles, and general connective tissues) are called
    a. carcinomas.
    b. lymphomas.
    c. leukemia.
    d. sarcomas.

11. A large group of diseases characterized by uncontrolled growth and spread of abnormal cells is called
    a. mutant cells.
    b. neoplasms.
    c. carcinogens.
    d. cancer.

12. Physicians who specialize in the treatment of malignancies are called
    a. oncologists.
    b. internists.
    c. cancerologists.
    d. epidemiologists.

13. Cancer of the epithelial tissues, in particular the breast, lungs, intestines, skin and mouth, are classified as
    a. carcinomas.
    b. sarcomas.
    c. lymphomas.
    d. leukemia.

14. One of the most common types of cancer, characterized by solid tumors, found in males between the ages of 17 and 34 is
    a. testicular cancer.
    b. prostate cancer.
    c. liver cancer.
    d. stomach cancer.

15. Carcinomas are
    a. cancer-causing agents.
    b. antigens found in the prostate of cancer patients.
    c. harmless, noncancerous tumors.
    d. suspected cancer-causing agents.

Practice Test #2

1. What is the leading cause of cancer death in women?
   a. breast cancer
   b. lung cancer
   c. cervical cancer
   d. ovarian cancer

2. What is the most common sign of ovarian cancer?
   a. weight gain
   b. unusual amounts of gas
   c. digestive irregularities
   d. enlarged abdomen

3. Hodgkin's disease is a type of
   a. leukemia.
   b. lymphoma.
   c. carcinoma.
   d. sarcoma.

4. Which of the following is a source of ionizing radiation?
   a. radon
   b. microwaves
   c. computer screens
   d. electric blankets

5. Cancer-causing genes that are present on chromosomes are called
   a. epigenes.
   b. oncogenes.
   c. primogenes.
   d. metastogenes.

6. Bleeding from the rectum, blood in the stool, and changes in bowel habits are the major warning signals for which type of cancer?
   a. kidney
   b. pancreatic
   c. colon and rectal
   d. breast

7. When breast and lymph nodes in the immediate area are removed, it is a
   a. lumpectomy.
   b. modified radical mastectomy.
   c. radical mastectomy.
   d. simple mastectomy.

8. What is most effective in treating localized cancer masses?
   a. radiotherapy
   b. chemotherapy
   c. surgery
   d. immunotherapy

9. The process by which cancer spreads from one area to other areas of the body is called
   a. mutation.
   b. ionization.
   c. metastasis.
   d. neoplasmic.

10. The deadly form of skin cancer that is the most frequent cancer in women ages 24 to 29 is
    a. basal cell skin cancer.
    b. malignant melanoma.
    c. squamous cell skin cancer.
    d. epithelial cell cancer.

11. A food additive suspected of causing cancer is
    a. sodium.
    b. diethylstilbestrol.
    c. nitrosamines.
    d. asbestos.

12. In general, ordinary-looking cells enclosed in a fibrous shell or capsule that prevents their spreading to other body areas are called
    a. mutant cells.
    b. malignant tumors.
    c. benign tumors.
    d. metastatic tumors.

13. Suspected cancer-causing genes present on chromosomes are called
    a. mutations.
    b. familial genes.
    c. oncogenes.
    d. prototype genes.

14. What are the most common occupational carcinogens?
    a. asbestos
    b. pesticides
    c. coal tars
    d. lead

15. A virulent cancer of the melanin portion of the skin that can be fatal and results from radiation from the sun is called
    a. multiple myelomas.
    b. malignant melanoma.
    c. Kaposi's sarcoma.
    d. basal cell carcinoma.

17 Infectious Diseases and Sexually Transmitted Infections

General Review Questions

1. What factors influence your susceptibility to diseases?
2. What are the routes that pathogens enter the body?
3. List and give an example of the major types of pathogens.
4. What are the body linings that provide protection against pathogens?
5. Who is the fastest-growing segment of the HIV population in the United States?

Practice Test #1

1. Organisms that normally live in coexistence with human hosts and are usually harmless are called
   a. pathogens.
   b. exogenous microorganisms.
   c. endogenous microorganisms.
   d. infections microorganisms.

2. In 1993 the city of Milwaukee experienced many deaths and illnesses and 4,500 hospitalizations due to a waterborne disease caused by an intestinal parasite called
   a. E. coli.
   b. hantavirus.
   c. cryptosporidium.
   d. ebola.

3. Any substance capable of triggering an immune response is called a(n)
   a. antibody.
   b. antigen.
   c. enzyme.
   d. prion.

4. A viral disorder which occurs mostly in children, causes swelling of the salivary glands, and can potentially lead to sterility in men is called
   a. mumps.
   b. chicken pox.
   c. measles.
   d. rabies.

5. A virally caused disease resulting in inflamation of the liver and characterized by symptoms including fever, loss of appetite and skin rashes is called
   a. hepatitis.
   b. mononucleosis.
   c. influenza.
   d. mumps.

6. Staphylococcal infection is a form of
   a. rickettsia infection.
   b. fungi infection.
   c. viral infection.
   d. bacterial infection.

7. The smallest of the pathogens is
   a. rickettsia.
   b. virus.
   c. parasitic worms.
   d. bacteria.

8. The body's single most critical early defense system to infection is
   a. cilia.
   b. t-lymphocytes.
   c. tears.
   d. skin.

9. White blood cells that aid in the antigen-antibody response are known as
   a. antigens.
   b. lymphocytes.
   c. phagocytes.
   d. erythrocytes.

10. The most commonly reported sexually transmitted infection (STI) in the United States is
    a. human papilloma virus.
    b. urinary tract infections.
    c. syphilis.
    d. genital herpes.

11. What inherited blood disease affects African Americans and results in organ damage and premature death?
a. AIDS
b. sickle cell anemia
c. diabetes
d. muscular dystrophy

12. Benny prefers his beef cooked very rare. What type of food-borne infection should he be concerned about?
a. Lyme disease
b. rabies
c. E. coli
d. botulism

13. The sexually transmitted infection that is characterized in males by a white milky discharge from the penis, along with painful, burning urination two to nine days after contact is
a. syphilis.
b. gonorrhea.
c. candidiasis.
d. genital warts.

14. The slow-acting virus that causes AIDS is
a. herpes simplex.
b. human papilloma virus.
c. human immunodeficiency virus.
d. neisseria gonorrhea.

15. Which of the following is *not* a major body fluid of concern for HIV?
a. blood
b. semen
c. saliva
d. vaginal secretions

Practice Test #2

1. Touching the handle of a towel dispenser that has just been touched by a person whose hands were contaminated by a sneeze is an example of
a. direct contact.
b. indirect contact.
c. food-borne transmission.
d. airborne transmission.

2. One fatal disease which was widespread in the U.S. in the early 1900s and then controlled in the mid-1900s only to be making a comeback now is
a. Legionnaire's disease.
b. pneumonia..
c. tuberculosis.
d. rickettsia.

3. Cocci, bacilli and spirilla are the three major types of
a. toxins.
b. staph infections.
c. streptococci.
d. bacteria.

4. When you transmit a pathogen from one part of your body to another, that is known as
a. autoinoculation.
b. interspecies trasmission.
c. self-transmission.
d. perinatal transmission

5. The single greatest factor influencing your longevity is your
a. immune system.
b. environment.
c. organism resistance.
d. parents' longevity.

6. The time between when an agent breaks through the body's defenses and the first appearance of symptoms is called the
a. infection period.
b. incubation period.
c. antibody period.
d. immune period.

7. A viral disease that causes inflammation of the liver is
a. hepatitis.
b. herpes simplex.
c. AIDS.
d. measles.

8. Single-celled organisms that cause diseases such as trichomoniasis and giardiasis are called
a. fungi.
b. bacteria.
c. rickettsia.
d. protozoa.

9. Which of the following infections is caused by fungi?
   a. ringworm
   b. trichomoniasis
   c. rabies
   d. pneumonia

10. Treatments that are administered orally or by injection for the purpose of forming an artificial immunity are called
    a. vaccinations.
    b. acquired immunity.
    c. natural immunity.
    d. passive immunity.

11. The stage of syphilis that is often characterized by the development of a sore known as a chancre is
    a. primary syphilis.
    b. secondary syphilis.
    c. latent syphilis.
    d. late syphilis.

12. Human papilloma viruses have been associated with increased risk of
    a. chancres.
    b. blistering sores or eruptions on the skin.
    c. cervical cancer.
    d. pelvic inflammatory disease.

13. In adults, the average length of time it takes HIV to cause slow, degenerative changes in the immune system is
    a. 4-6 years.
    b. 8-10 years.
    c. 11-13 years.
    d. 15 years or longer.

14. The blood test used to detect the presence of HIV antibodies is the
    a. ELISA.
    b. HIV antibody test.
    c. HIV-1 immunoassay.
    d. colposcopy.

15. One of the most widespread sexually transmitted infections in the world is
    a. HIV infection.
    b. genital herpes.
    c. genital warts.
    d. trichomoniasis.

18 Noninfectious Conditions

General Review Questions

1. What are the most common environmental antigens that cause responses for allergy-induced problems?
2. List the "five f's" of gallbladder disease risk.
3. List the risk factors for low back pain.
4. What are the criteria for diagnosing chronic fatigue syndrome?
5. What injuries can result from repetitive stress injury?

Practice Test #1

1. A respiratory disease in which the alveoli of the lungs are gradually destroyed is called
   a. asthma.
   b. hay fever.
   c. emphysema.
   d. chronic bronchitis.

2. What is the most common chronic disease of childhood?
   a. asthma
   b. bronchitis
   c. rheumatic fever
   d. streptococcal infection

3. What is the hallmark of Parkinson's disease?
   a. tremors
   b. poor balance
   c. slurred speech
   d. rigidity in the muscles

4. Symptoms for diabetes include all of the following, *except*
   a. excessive thirst.
   b. hypoglycemia.
   c. frequent urination.
   d. skin eruptions.

5. Type-1 Diabetes is
   a. adult-onset diabetes.
   b. non-insulin dependent.
   c. developed later in life.
   d. insulin-dependent.

6. When the gallbladder has been repeatedly irritated and reduces its ability to release bile, what disease can result?
   a. diverticulosis
   b. colitis
   c. cholecystitis
   d. appendicitis

7. Rheumatoid arthritis is
   a. a progressive deterioration of the bones and joints.
   b. affected by weather changes, excessive strain and injury.
   c. an autoimmune disorder that attacks the synovial membrane which produces the lubricating fluids of the joint.
   d. caused by abnormal use of the joint and abnormalities in joint structure.

8. The risk of low back pain can be reduced by all of the following, *except*
   a. exercises that strengthen stomach muscles.
   b. maintaining good posture.
   c. sleeping on your stomach.
   d. stretching the back muscles.

9. A syndrome describing a series of characteristic symptoms that occur prior to menstruation in some women is
   a. endometriosis.
   b. fibrocystic breast condition.
   c. premenstrual syndrome.
   d. diabetes.

10. A common repetitive stress injury associated with typing at the computer and resulting in irriation to the median nerve in the wrist is called
    a. carpal tunnel syndrome.
    b. chronic fatigue syndrome.
    c. chronic Epstein Barr disease.
    d. seasonal affective disorder.

11. Chemical substances that dilate blood vessels, increase mucous secretions, cause tissues to swell, and produce other allergy-like symptoms are called
   a. allergens.
   b. antibodies.
   c. histamines.
   d. antigens.

12. What is a major cause of exercise-induced asthma?
   a. cold, dry air
   b. ragweed and flower blooms
   c. animal dander
   d. mold

13. What seizure disorder is characterized by no convulsions, minor loss of consciousness that may go unnoticed, and a minor twitching of muscles?
   a. Jacksonian seizure
   b. gand mal seizure
   c. petit mal seizure
   d. psychomotor seizure

14. Diverticulosis occurs when
   a. the intestinal walls become inflamed.
   b. the intestinal walls become weakened for undetermined reasons and small pea-shaped bulges develop.
   c. the pancreas fails to produce enough insulin.
   d. endometrial tissue develops abnormally outside the uterus.

15. All of the following are common treatments for PMS, *except*
   a. aspirin for pain.
   b. stress reduction techniques.
   c. exercise.
   d. decreased intake of complex carbohydrates.

Practice Test #2

1. What is the most common type of asthma?
   a. intrinsic
   b. extrinsic
   c. exercise-induced
   d. food intolerance

2. Which of the following is *not* a neurological disorder?
   a. headaches
   b. multiple sclerosis
   c. Parkinson's disease
   d. diabetes

3. A degenerative neurological disease in which the myelin breaks down and causes nerve malfunction is called
   a. cerebral palsy.
   b. multiple sclerosis.
   c. Parkinson's disease.
   d. Grave's disease.

4. Women with menstrual cycles shorter than 27 days and those with flows lasting over a week are at increased risk for
   a. endometriosis.
   b. premenstrual syndrome.
   c. cervical cancer.
   d. ovarian cancer.

5. Anyone who is female, fat, fair, forty, and flatulent appears to be at increased risk for
   a. gallbladder disease.
   b. ulcerative colitis.
   c. peptic ulcers.
   d. diverticulosis.

6. Headaches that arise as a result of some other underlying condition, such as hyptertension, are known as what type of headache?
   a. tension
   b. secondary
   c. migraine
   d. psychsomatic

7. Which of the following is *not* a COPD?
   a. asthma
   b. diabetes
   c. emphysema
   d. chronic bronchitis

8. In what part of the country are people most prone to asthma?
   a. East
   b. Midwest
   c. South
   d. West

9. What chronic respiratory disease is characterized by attacks of wheezing, shortness of breath and coughing spasms?
   a. allergies
   b. asthma
   c. emphysema
   d. chronic bronchitis

10. What is the typical cause of chronic bronchitis?
   a. ragweed and pollen
   b. use of cigarettes
   c. animal dander
   d. dust

11. What is a common noncancerous problem among women in the United States?
   a. fibrocystic breast condition
   b. petit mal seizures
   c. colitis
   d. diverticulosis

12. Hyperglycemia refers to
   a. excessive thirst.
   b. increased appetite.
   c. elevated blood sugars.
   d. increased urinary output.

13. Some peptic ulcers are believed to be caused by
   a. inflammation of the intestinal walls.
   b. the weakening of intestinal walls for undetermined reasons and the development of small pea-shaped bulges,
   c. the inability of the pancreas to produce enough insulin,
   d. the erosive effect of digestive juices on the lining of the stomach or the duodenum,

14. A condition of repetitive cessation of breathing during sleep that can lead to dramatic rises in blood pressure is called
   a. sleep apnea.
   b. chronic bronchitis.
   c. lupus.
   d. emphysema.

15. A butterfly-shaped rash covering the bridge of the nose and both cheeks is a common symptom of
   a. chronic fatigue syndrome.
   b. Raynaud's syndrome.
   c. scleroderma.
   d. lupus.

19 Healthy Aging

General Review Questions

1. Describe the two psychosocial theories of personality development that encompass the human life span.
2. What are the estimated health care costs of the elderly?
3. List the risk factors for osteoporosis.
4. How is intelligence affected by age?
5. What does it mean to age successfully?

Practice Test #1

1. The study of the individual and collective aging process is called
   a. ageology.
   b. gerontology.
   c. genealogy.
   d. archeology.

2. Age-associated loss of muscle mass is also known as
   a. sarcopenia.
   b. osteoporosis.
   c. comorbidity.
   d. glaucoma.

3. What percentage of elderly people live in a nursing home at some point in their life?
   a. 5%
   b. 33%
   c. 50%
   d. 70%

4. According to Erik Erikson,
   a. people must progress through eight critical stages during their lifetime.
   b. painful aging is caused by a lack of appropriate coping skills.
   c. aging is related to the amount of mutational damage within the genes.
   d. as we age our immune systems become more effective in fighting disease.

5. As the aging process continues, the loss of calcium and loss of minerals can affect
   a. the skin.
   b. bones and joints.
   c. heart and lungs.
   d. the urinary tract.

6. A person's habits and roles relative to society's expectations refers to his or her
   a. functional age.
   b. psychological age.
   c. legal age.
   d. social age.

7. A term used to describe loss of memory and judgment and orientation problems occurring in a small percentage of the elderly is
   a. senility.
   b. depression.
   c. psychosis.
   d. schizophrenia.

8. One of the most common forms of dementia for the elderly is
   a. Alzheimer's disease.
   b. incontinence.
   c. depression.
   d. psychosis.

9. The "young-old" are people who are
   a. 55-64 years of age.
   b. 65-74 years of age.
   c. 75-84 years of age.
   d. 85 years or older.

10. According to the cellular theory, aging is caused by
    a. the human body wearing out.
    b. the body's cells having reached the end of their reproductive cycle.
    c. the decline of the body's immunological system.
    d. an increased number of cells exhibiting unusual or different characteristics with increased age.

11. A clouding of the eye lens is called
   a. cataracts.
   b. glaucoma.
   c. colorblindness.
   d. astigmatism.

12. During menopause, women may experience
   a. hot flashes.
   b. weight gain.
   c. the development of facial hair.
   d. all of the above

13. Your grandmother has suddenly been acting strange. She has been disoriented, erratic, and cannot make a cup of coffee. What may be causing her to behave so strangely?
   a. She may be developing an age-related disorder (i.e., dementia).
   b. She may be having an adverse reaction to OTC drugs.
   c. She may be having an adverse reaction to a prescription medication.
   d. All of the above

14. The inability to control urination is called
   a. osteoporosis.
   b. vital capacity.
   c. urinary incontinence.
   d. None of the above

15. A chronic condition involving changes in nerve fibers of the brain that results in mental deterioration is called
   a. Alzheimer's disease.
   b. presenile dementia.
   c. Parkinson's disease.
   d. senility.

Practice Test #2

1. The patterns of life changes that occur in members of all species as they grow older is called
   a. aging.
   b. gerontology.
   c. maturity.
   d. maturation.

2. What is the cause of Alzheimer's disease?
   a. neurotransmitter imbalance
   b. malfunction of the immune system
   c. slow-acting virus
   d. currently unknown

3. What nutrient is necessary for adequate calcium absorption?
   a. Vitamin D
   b. Vitamin K
   c. Vitamin B
   d. Vitamin E

4. In 2000, there were 35 million Americans age 65 or older. By 2030, this number will be
   a. 50 million.
   b. 60 million.
   c. 70 million.
   d. 80 million.

5. The life expectancy for a person born in 1998 is
   a. 63 years.
   b. 68 years.
   c. 72 years.
   d. 77 years.

6. What is the most common definition of age in the United States?
   a. biological age
   b. social age
   c. legal age
   d. functional age

7. What percent of all people between the ages of 65 and 74 are forced to seek nursing-home care?
   a. 1%
   b. 15%
   c. 20%
   d. 40%

8. According to the autoimmune theory, aging is caused by
   a. the human body wearing out.
   b. the body's cells having reached the end of their reproductive cycle.
   c. the decline of the body's immunological system.
   d. an increased number of cells exhibiting unusual or different characteristics with increased age.

9. The elevation of pressure within the eyeball that can lead to blindness is called
   a. cataracts.
   b. glaucoma.
   c. far-sightedness.
   d. near-sightedness.

10. Elderly people are at increased risk of hypothermia, heat stroke, and heat exhaustion because
    a. pain receptors are more sensitive.
    b. there is a loss of body fat.
    c. tactile senses improve.
    d. the skin becomes thicker.

11. Prevention of osteoporosis focuses on
    a. maintaining muscular strength and flexibility.
    b. daily weight bearing exercise.
    c. adequate calcium intake.
    d. All of the above

12. Based on a recent study by the National Council on Aging,
    a. most older american males cannot have sexual intercourse.
    b. nearly half of americans over the age of 60 engage in sexual activity at least once a month.
    c. most older american women do not want to have sexual intercourse.
    d. most older american females cannot have sexual intercourse due to the physical changes from menopause.

13. Elderly women are more likely to need assistance from their children, other relatives, friends, and neighbors than men because
    a. there are more elderly women than men.
    b. women do not age as well as men.
    c. women have more serious health problems (i.e. osteoporosis) than men.
    d. men are the primary caregivers.

14. What are the most commonly used over-the-counter drugs among the elderly?
    a. aspirin and laxatives
    b. vitamin supplements
    c. Geritol and One-a-Day vitamins
    d. antacids and laxatives

15. What country has the highest percentage of their population that is 60 years of age and over?
    a. Uruguay
    b. United States
    c. France
    d. Italy

20 Dying and Death

General Review Questions

1. How is death determined by the Uniform Determination of Death Act?
2. What factors influence our attitudes about death?
3. List the five stages of dying.
4. What are the arguments for and against PAS?
5. What artificial life support techniques may be legally refused by competent patients in some states?

Practice Test #1

1. Dying is defined as
   a. the final cessation of the vital functions of the body.
   b. an irreversible situation in which a person is laid to rest.
   c. the process of decline in body functions resulting in the death of an organism.
   d. the cessation of electrical activity in the brain.

2. Events like a divorce that resemble death in that they involve separation, termination and a change in self-perception are called
   a. quasi-death experiences.
   b. near-death experiences.
   c. grief experiences.
   d. life-and-death experiences.

3. The dying are placed in huts that will later be burned. After they die, mourners wear wreaths of green leaves and cut themselves with knives. This is the practice
   a. in China.
   b. among Muslims in the Middle East.
   c. among the Maori of New Zealand.
   d. in Judaism.

4. Which of the following statements is true concerning men and women who have recently lost a spouse?
   a. Men show more emotion to other people.
   b. Men felt the funeral process was important.
   c. Men tended to remarry sooner.
   d. Men usually expressed more concern about the cost of the funeral.

5. The process of accepting the reality of a person's death and coping with memories of the deceased is called
   a. grief.
   b. grief work.
   c. disenfranchised grief.
   d. mourning.

6. Brain death occurs when
   a. there is no response even to painful stimuli.
   b. there is no movement for a continuous hour after observation by a physician and no breathing after three minutes off a respirator.
   c. the pupils are fixed and dilated.
   d. All of the above

7. Angela's grandmother is dying but she keeps assuring her sisters that their grandmother will be and will be coming home soon. Angela is most likely experiencing
   a. grief.
   b. mourning.
   c. death denial.
   d. bereavement.

8. The stage of grief that is characterized by the dying person resolving to be a better person in return for an extension of life is called
   a. denial.
   b. anger.
   c. bargaining.
   d. depression.

9. An irreversible situation in which a person is not treated like an active member of society is called
   a. local death.
   b. functional death.
   c. social death.
   d. somatic death.

10. Bereavement is
    a. mental distress caused by a loss that cannot be openly acknowledged, publicly mourned, or socially supported.
    b. loss or deprivation experienced by a survivor when a loved one dies.
    c. a culturally sanctioned display of grief.
    d. mental distress that occurs in reaction to the loss of a loved one.

11. Extramarital lovers who find it difficult to mourn the death of their lover because of societal stigmas may experience
    a. bereavement.
    b. bereavement displacement.
    c. disenfranchised grief.
    d. denial.

12. Saul has experienced many losses in his life, including the loss of his wife, friends, and children. His gloomy outlook and disturbing behavior patterns may be symptomatic of
    a. an age-associated dementia.
    b. self-pity.
    c. bereavement overload.
    d. depression.

13. May has not dated anyone for the past year since her fiancée died and has visited his grave every week. Her actions may be described as
    a. mourning.
    b. grief.
    c. death affiliation.
    d. death expectations.

14. Funerals serve the purpose of
    a. maximizing the quality of life of the survivors.
    b. relieving a dying person' pain.
    c. assisting survivors of the deceased in coping with their loss.
    d. keeping the memory of the deceased alive to the family and friends.

15. The type of "mercy-killing" which is accomplished by administering large doses of painkillers that depress the central nervous system to the extent that basic life-sustaining regulatory centers cease to function is called
    a. suicide.
    b. active euthanasia.
    c. passive euthanasia.
    d. dyathanasia.

Practice Test #2

1. The view that death is the "mortal enemy of mankind" reflects
    a. death acceptance.
    b. death denial.
    c. death procrastination.
    d. death avoidance.

2. The decision of a terminally ill person to kill herself rather than endure constant pain is called
    a. active euthanasia.
    b. rational suicide.
    c. physician-assisted death.
    d. resuscitation.

3. Someone who dies without a will is said to be
    a. interstate.
    b. intrastate.
    c. intrastate.
    d. interstitual.

4. The mental state of distress that occurs in reaction to significant loss is called
    a. grief.
    b. disenfranchised grief.
    c. mourning.
    d. bereavement.

5. After the death of a family member, other family members do not shave, bathe, wear leather shes or get haircuts. This is the practice
    a. in China.
    b. among Muslims in the Middle East.
    c. among the Maori of New Zealand.
    d. in Judaism.

6. The funeral visitation provides a(n)
    a. chance for the family to visit with friends and loved ones.
    b. time and place for friends to offer their expression of sorrow and sympathy.
    c. opportunity for friends and loved ones to see the flowers and cards sent to the family.
    d. opportunity for friends and loved ones to specify what charitable organization they sent a donation to in the deceased's name.

7. The form of "mercy killing" in which life-prolonging treatments or interventions are not offered or withheld, thereby allowing a terminally ill person to die naturally is called
   a. self-deliverance.
   b. euthanasia.
   c. dyathanasia.
   d. suicide.

8. The stage of grief in which vitality diminishes and the patient begins to experience distress symptoms with increasing frequency is called
   a. denial.
   b. bargaining.
   c. depression.
   d. acceptance.

9. Bereavement overload occurs when
   a. there is the loss of a loved one that cannot be openly acknowledged or publicly mourned.
   b. the loss is a significant loved one.
   c. there are multiple losses and the accumulating sorrow in the lives of some elderly people.
   d. the survivor experiences significant physical and mental distress.

10. After her husband died, Sue began to experience a loss of appetite, an inability to sleep at night, and was unable to concentrate. She may be experiencing
    a. bereavement.
    b. mourning.
    c. denial.
    d. grief.

11. Grief work is
    a. the process of integrating the reality of the loss with everyday life and learning to feel better.
    b. the total acceptance that a loved one has died.
    c. assigning feelings to the loss of a loved one.
    d. completing the cultural rituals that are required to express one's grief.

12. To help children cope, it is important to
    a. give children the opportunity to attend the funeral.
    b. encourage the expression of feelings.
    c. provide convincing assurance that there will be somebody to love and look after the child.
    d. All of the above

13. All of the following are characteristics of hospice programs, *except*
    a. services are provided by only specially trained nurses.
    b. emphasis is placed on symptom control, primarily the alleviation of pain.
    c. coverage is provided 24 hours a day, seven days per week.
    d. care of the family extends through the bereavement period.

14. While people react differently to losses,
    a. most people experience a release of joy when a loved one dies.
    b. few people have physical symptoms in response to their loss.
    c. people who have a stronger social support system tend to progress through the progression of grief more smoothly.
    d. most people recall all of the good and bad things that the deceased did to them.

15. Kerri's grandmother is been very sick and wants to die. Her family has agreed to withhold treatment that may prolong her life. This is called
    a. rational suicide.
    b. self-deliverance.
    c. passive euthanasia.
    d. active euthanasia.

21 Environmental Health

General Review Questions

1. What environmental concerns arise as global population continues to expand?
2. List the six primary sources of indoor air pollution.
3. What are the global environmental consequences of rapid deforestation in Central and South America, Africa, and Southeast Asia?
4. What are the sources of nonpoint pollution?
5. List three ways that our society can manage solid waste.

Practice Test #1

1. Sulfur dioxide, a yellowish-brown gas, can
   a. aggravate heart and lung disease.
   b. corrode metals.
   c. impair visibility.
   d. All of the above

2. What is the principle source of hydrocarbons?
   a. automobile engines
   b. industrial paints
   c. coal-burning plants
   d. All of the above

3. What weather condition occurs when a layer of cool air is trapped under a layer of warmer air and prevents the air from circulating?
   a. Greenhouse effect
   b. ozone
   c. temperature inversion
   d. photochemical smog

4. What substance separates into stringy fibers, lodges in lungs and can cause lung cancer?
   a. asbestos
   b. particulate matter
   c. radon
   d. formaldehyde

5. The odorless, colorless gas that originates primarily from motor vehicle emissions and interferes wit the blood's ability to absorb oxygen is called
   a. sulfur dioxide.
   b. carbon monoxide.
   c. nitrogen dioxide.
   d. ozone.

6. What country is projected to have the largest increase in population by the year 2050?
   a. India
   b. United States
   c. Zimbabwe
   d. Mexico

7. Premature puberty in girls, genital defects in boys and rapidly falling sperm counts in men may be the result of alterations caused by organic compounds with chlorine attached called
   a. endocrine disrupting chemicals (EDCs).
   b. particulates.
   c. chlorofluorocarbons (CFCs).
   d. heavy metals.

8. Chlorofluorocarbons, chemicals that contribute to the depletion of the ozone layer, are found in
   a. refrigerators.
   b. air conditioners.
   c. various foam products.
   d. All of the above

9. How much of the earth is covered with water?
   a. 15%
   b. 45%
   c. 60%
   d. 75%

10. Which of the following is an example of a point source pollutant?
    a. soil erosion
    b. leakage from septic tanks
    c. pesticide runoff
    d. releases from a sewage treatment plant

11. One cause of steep decline in public support for nuclear power was a 1979 accident at a Pennsylvania nuclear facility called
    a. Chernobyl.
    b. Three Mile Island.
    c. Indian Point.
    d. Fermi.

12. Industrial chemicals that can cause cancer and are used in high voltage electrical equipment, such as transformers, are known as
   a. dioxins.
   b. polychlorinated biphenyls (PCBs).
   c. pesticides.
   d. trichlorethylene (TCE).

13. Municipal solid waste contains
   a. containers and packaging.
   b. durable goods.
   c. industrial wastes.
   d. All of the above

14. The recommended maximum "safe" dosage of radiation is
   a. 0.5 rads to 5 rads per year.
   b. 2.5 rads to 35 rads per year.
   c. 50 rads to 60 rads per year.
   d. 100 rads to 200 rads per year.

15. Radiation produced by photons having energy high enough to ionize atoms is called
   a. radioactive emissions.
   b. nuclear energy.
   c. fission.
   d. ionizing radiation.

Practice Test #2

1. What is the most predominant greenhouse gas?
   a. lead
   b. formaldehyde
   c. carbon dioxide
   d. chlorofluorocarbons

2. A six-year study by the National Institute of Environmental Health Sciences concluded that the evidence of a link between cancer and electric and magnetic fields (EMFs) is
   a. weak.
   b. inconclusive.
   c. strong.
   d. irrefutable.

3. The most common way to detect gasoline in the water supply is to test for
   a. benzene.
   b. leachate.
   c. PCBs.
   d. dioxins.

4. One source of indoor pollution which can produce cancer is a strong-smelling gas present in some draperies and carpets called
   a. radon.
   b. asbestos.
   c. formaldehyde.
   d. ozone.

5. The United Nations projects that the world population will grow from 6.1 billion in 2000 to a population in the year 2050 of
   a. 6.8 billion.
   b. 7.4 billion.
   c. 9.4 billion.
   d. 12.4 billion.

6. The bulk of population growth is in
   a. Eastern Europe.
   b. developing countries in urban areas.
   c. the South American rain forests.
   d. the United States.

7. The single biggest contributor towards zero population growth is
   a. institutionalized birth control with methods.
   b. mass sterilization.
   c. education.
   d. abortion.

8. The single greatest source of acid rain in the United States is
   a. coal-fired power plants.
   b. motor vehicle exhaust.
   c. chemical pollutants.
   d. wood stove smoke.

9. Exposure to formaldehyde can cause which of the following health problems?
   a. respiratory problems
   b. fatigue
   c. cancer
   d. All of the above

10. Chemicals that are designed to kill insects, rodents, plants, and fungi are called
   a. pesticides.
   b. polychlorinated biphenyls.
   c. dioxins.
   d. benzene.

11. Chemicals that contribute to the depletion of the ozone layer are called
    a. ozone.
    b. chlorofluorocarbons.
    c. hydrocarbons.
    d. carbon monoxide.

12. Which of the following is *not* a greenhouse gas?
    a. carbon dioxide
    b. radon
    c. ground level ozone
    d. methane

13. The two major categories of point source pollutants are
    a. sewage treatment plants and landfills.
    b. sewage treatment plants and industrial facilities.
    c. acid mine leakage and landfills.
    d. industrial facilities and landfills.

14. Long-term exposure to pesticides has been linked to
    a. birth defects.
    b. liver and kidney damage.
    c. nervous system disorders.
    d. All of the above

15. Which of the following is a symptom of noise-related distress?
    a. decreased blood pressure
    b. increased productivity
    c. decreased cholesterol levels
    d. increased secretion of adrenaline

22 Consumerism

General Review Questions

1. Differentiate between nonprofit and proprietary hospitals.
2. What are examples of common ambulatory facilities?
3. List the major problems with the health care system that have led to change.
4. How do prescription drugs become OTC drugs?
5. Describe the three major types of HMOs.

Practice Test #1

1. What is the single greatest difficulty that we face as health care consumers?
   a. The limited number of physicians who will accept new patients.
   b. Being reimbursed by insurance companies and limited coverage.
   c. The sheer magnitude of choices available to consumers.
   d. Not knowing the adverse and often unforeseeable effects of medical treatments.

2. Eduardo's back pain disappears in five days without any treatment. This is an example of
   a. disease prevention.
   b. the placebo effect.
   c. spontaneous remission.
   d. complementary medical treatment.

3. The number of emergency room visits has decreased dramatically in recent years due mostly to
   a. managed care.
   b. Americans becoming more healthy.
   c. the closing of many emergency rooms.
   d. the decreasing cost of emergency room care.

4. What drugs are used to kill or stop bacteria growth?
   a. analgesics
   b. antibiotics
   c. sedatives
   d. tranquilizers

5. What drugs are central nervous system depressants that induce sleep and relieve anxiety?
   a. analgesics
   b. antibiotics
   c. amphetamines
   d. sedatives

6. A medical practitioner who treats routine ailments, advises on preventive care, gives general medical advice, and makes appropriate referrals when necessary is called a
   a. general practitioner.
   b. family primary provider.
   c. primary care practitioner.
   d. primary family physician.

7. In what type of HMO system does a patient receive care from salaried staff doctors at the HMO's only facility?
   a. staff model
   b. group network model
   c. group intervention association
   d. independent practice association

8. A midlevel practitioner trained to handle most standard cases of care is a
   a. physician's assistant.
   b. nurse practitioner.
   c. licensed practical nurse.
   d. nurse.

9. Medical alternatives to traditional medicine are known as
   a. allopathic medicine.
   b. primary medicine.
   c. nonallopathic medicine.
   d. chiropractic medicine.

10. Treatments or services that do not require an overnight stay in a hospital are called
    a. ambulatory care.
    b. proprietary services.
    c. outpatient care.
    d. both a and c

11. When a private hospital (for-profit) hospital transfers a patient who is unable to pay to a public hospital, this is called
   a. skimming.
   b. patient dumping.
   c. GOMERS.
   d. bumping.

12. Hospitals run by religious or other humanitarian groups that reinvest their earnings in the hospital to improve health care are called
   a. health maintenance organizations.
   b. outpatient care centers.
   c. for-profit hospitals.
   d. nonprofit hospitals.

13. Medicaid provides coverage for
   a. elderly over 65 years of age.
   b. all people total and permanently disabled.
   c. all people with end-stage renal failure.
   d. All of the above

14. Physicians who belong to a Preferred Provider Organization
   a. usually reimbursed on a discounted fee-for-service basis.
   b. do not need to participate in utilization reviews.
   c. must restrict their practice to only patients on the insurance plan.
   d. are only reimbursed at 50-60% of the cost of services.

15. Rosa is a college student who works part-time and has limited health insurance through her student fees. She only makes about $13,000 a year. If she has to have her appendix removed, it could cost about $7,000. At this point in her life, Rosa
   a. is not insured.
   b. is underinsured.
   c. is overinsured.
   d. doesn't need insurance.

Practice Test #2

1. Amanda is having trouble seeing and needs to have new glasses. She would most likely visit an
   a. orthodontist.
   b. optometrist.
   c. ophthalmologist.
   d. orthopedist.

2. As a result of an automobile accident, Huang had a broken jaw that will require extensive surgical procedures. He will most likely need to see a(n)
   a. dentist.
   b. orthodontist.
   c. orthopedic surgeon.
   d. oral surgeon.

3. The largest sales category of over-the-counter drugs in the United States, with $2 billion in sales, is
   a. analgesics.
   b. stimulants.
   c. sleeping aids.
   d. dieting aids.

4. The interaction of two or more drugs in which the effects of the individual drugs are multiplied is called
   a. antagonism.
   b. synergism.
   c. inhibition.
   d. intolerance.

5. General practitioners who receive training similar to a medical doctor but who emphasize the skeletal and muscular systems are called
   a. nurses.
   b. physician assistants.
   c. osteopaths.
   d. opthamologists.

6. Alice has health insurance but has to spend more than 10% of her income on medical care because her insurance is inadequate. She is
   a. uninsured.
   b. underinsured.
   c. overinsured.
   d. reinsured.

7. Informed consent is the right to have understandable information about
   a. side effects of the medical treatment.
   b. benefits of the medical treatment.
   c. available options to the medical treatment.
   d. All of the above

8. A medical practice based on scientifically validated methods and procedures whose objective is to heal by countering the patient's symptoms is considered
   a. allopathic medicine.
   b. nonallopathic medicine.
   c. osteopathic medicine.
   d. chiropractic medicine.

9. Herbal medicine, massage, megavitamins, and energy healing are all types of
   a. allopathic medicine.
   b. placebos.
   c. complementary medicine.
   d. chiropractic medicine.

10. Hospitals that provide a return on earnings to the investors who own them are called
    a. group practices.
    b. nonprofit hospitals.
    c. for-profit hospitals.
    d. ambulatory care centers.

11. In recent years, how much of the gross domestic produce (GDP) has been spent on health care?
    a. 5%
    b. 15%
    c. 20%
    d. 35%

12. A Chinese medical treatment that has been shown to improve quality of life and improve or cure certain health conditions is called
    a. massage.
    b. accupressure.
    c. homeopathy.
    d. herbal medicine.

13. A type of health insurance that provides a wide range of covered health benefits for a fixed amount prepaid by the employee, employer, or Medicare is called a
    a. prepaid group practice.
    b. health maintenance organization.
    c. preferred provider organization.
    d. public plan insurance.

14. Ophthalmologists specialize in the medical and surgical care of
    a. the eyes.
    b. the heart and blood vessels.
    c. the female reproductive system.
    d. cancerous growths and tumors.

15. The type of medical practice in which a group of physicians combine resources, sharing offices, equipment, and staff costs is called
    a. solo practice.
    b. group practice.
    c. fee-for-service practice.
    d. for-profit practice.

23 Complementary and Alternative Medicine

General Review Questions

1. What are the major types of CAM treatments?
2. What are the most sought-after forms of supplements on the market?
3. What exercise-related treatments are available?
4. What is the purpose of the German Commission E?
5. Who typically uses complementary and alternative medicine?

Practice Test #1

1. Functional foods are also known as
   a. phytomedicines.
   b. ergogenic aids.
   c. neutraceuticals.
   d. Ayurvedic medicine.

2. What percent of all modern pharmaceutical drugs are derived from herbs?
   a. 3%
   b. 10%
   c. 25%
   d. 47%

3. Ayurvedic medicine is a method of treatment derived greatly from ancient
   a. India.
   b. China.
   c. Japan.
   d. Egypt.

4. What system of diagnosis and treatment is based on history, an observation of the body, on palpitation, and on pulse diagnosis?
   a. acupuncture
   b. Ayurvedic medicine
   c. naturopathic treatment
   d. traditional Chinese medicine

5. Users of acupuncture are typically
   a. women.
   b. young adults, students, and blue-collar workers.
   c. middle-aged, well-educated, employed, and middle-income.
   d. middle-aged, well-educated, retired, and high-income.

6. If you believe that illness results from violations of natural principles of life in modern societies, you are a
   a. massage therapist.
   b. reflexologist.
   c. naturopath.
   d. iridologist.

7. Light therapy is also known as
   a. aromatherapy.
   b. auramassage.
   c. iridology.
   d. reflexology.

8. An ancient breathing and focusing exercise program, with exercises called *pranayama*, is called
   a. Tai Chi.
   b. yoga.
   c. body work.
   d. shiatsu.

9. A system of movements, floor exercises, and body work designed to retrain the central nervous system to help it find new pathways around any areas of blockage or damage is called
   a. shiatsu.
   b. yoga.
   c. Tai Chi.
   d. feldenkrais.

10. What is the main action of ginkgo?
    a. body builder
    b. blood thinner
    c. immune stimulator
    d. circulation enhancer

11. Echinacea is said to
    a. alleviate depression.
    b. improve short-term memory.
    c. fight motion sickness.
    d. stimulate the immune system.

12. The German Commission E attempts to
    a. educate the public about CAM.
    b. regulate the sale of alternative medicines and supplements.
    c. regulate CAM practitioners.
    d. challenge the popularity of CAM.

13. Different therapies based on the philosophy that humans produce waves of energy that are disrupted during illness defines
    a. iridology.
    b. energy healing.
    c. auromassage.
    d. reflexology.

14. Aloe, buckthorn, cascara, flaxseet, manna, psyllium, and senna leaf are all herbal remedies for
    a. constipation.
    b. memory loss.
    c. sleep disturbances.
    d. menopausal symptoms.

15. What special supplement is reported to have sexual restorative value?
    a. ginseng
    b. SAMe
    c. glucosamine
    d. chromium picolinate

Practice Test #2

1. What type of treatment uses substances and forces found in nature, such as crystals and minerals?
   a. naturopathic treatment
   b. iridology
   c. reflexology
   d. feldenkrais

2. An ancient exercise program that has been called "moving meditation" is called
   a. Tai Chi.
   b. yoga.
   c. feldenkrais.
   d. shiatsu.

3. What traditional healing art from Japan makes use of firm finger pressure applied to specific points on the body and is intended to increase the circulation of vital energy?
   a. shiatsu
   b. Tai Chi
   c. yoga
   d. acupressure

4. What herbal remedy has been shown to improve short-term memory?
   a. St. John's wort
   b. ginkgo biloba
   c. echinacea
   d. aloe

5. What herbal remedy seems to improve depression?
   a. echinacea
   b. ginkgo biloba
   c. St. John's wort
   d. soy protein

6. Compounds such as bee pollen, caffeine, glycine, and gelatin are typical forms of
   a. neutraceuticals.
   b. ergogenic aids.
   c. antioxidants.
   d. phytomedicines.

7. What substance manufactured by the body plays a key role in the growth and development of cartilage?
   a. ginseng
   b. creatine
   c. chromium picolinate
   d. glucosamine

8. Betacarotene, selenium, vitamin C, and vitamin E are primary
   a. neutraceuticals.
   b. antioxidants.
   c. ergogenic aids.
   d. phytomedicines.

9. What prebiotic fights motion sickness?
   a. ginger
   b. oat fiber
   c. soy protein
   d. yogurt

10. Medicinal herbs, many of which are sold over the counter in Europe, are also called
    a. ergogenic aids.
    b. neutraceuticals.
    c. tinctures.
    d. phytomedicines.

11. Individuals who seek alternative medicine over traditional allopathic medicine do so for the following reasons, *except*
    a. philosophical congruence.
    b. dissatisfaction with treatment.
    c. need for personal control.
    d. negative attitude toward traditional medicine.

12. Which of the following statements characterizing CAM users is *true*?
    a. Men are more likely to use CAM than women.
    b. Women are more likely to use CAM than men.
    c. Those with poorer health status are more likely to use CAM.
    d. Those with better health status are more likely to use CAM.

13. Two popular "treatments" that are supposed remedies for depression are
    a. gingko biloba and St. John's wort.
    b. gingko biloba and echinacea.
    c. St. John's wort and Kava.
    d. St. John's wort and echinacea.

14. What is the most frequently cited health problem treated with alternative therapies?
    a. arthritis
    b. headaches
    c. sprains
    d. chronic pain

15. Ginkgo biloba is used to treat
    a. constipation.
    b. memory loss.
    c. premenstrual syndrome.
    d. sleep disturbances.

Appendix A Injury Prevention and Emergency Care

General Review Questions

1. What is the "Good Samaritan Law?"
2. What are the symptoms of internal bleeding?
3. What population is at greatest risk of poisoning?
4. When does frostbite generally occur?
5. List the symptoms of hypothermia.

Practice Test #1

1. Which of the following questions should you be prepared to answer when calling for emergency assistance?
   a. Where are you and the victim located?
   b. Do you know the victim's name?
   c. What is the victim's apparent condition?
   d. All of the above

2. If a victim is unconscious,
   a. you must obtain the victim's consent in writing before administering first aid.
   b. you must make every reasonable effort to persuade the victim to accept your help.
   c. in emergency situations, consent is implied.
   d. you should wait until the victim regains consciousness to obtain consent.

3. Unintentional injuries are the leading cause of death for Americans
   a. over the age of 65.
   b. between the ages of 55-65.
   c. between the ages of 45-55.
   d. under the age of 45.

4. Failure to expel an obstructed object and restore breathing can lead to death in
   a. 30 seconds.
   b. 2 minutes.
   c. 6 minutes.
   d. 12 minutes.

5. The most effective method for assisting a choking victim is
   a. abdominal thrusts.
   b. Heimlich maneuver.
   c. rescue breathing.
   d. cardiopulmonary resuscitation.

6. If you suspect that someone is suffering from internal bleeding, which of the following steps should you take?
   a. Have the person lie on a flat surface with knees bent.
   b. Keep the victim warm.
   c. Do not give the victim any medications or fluids.
   d. All of the above

7. Victims of shock display all of the following symptoms, *except*
   a. dilated pupils.
   b. dry, hot skin.
   c. vomiting.
   d. delayed or unrelated responses to questions.

8. The majority of poisonings reported in the United States each year are caused by
   a. household products.
   b. gasoline.
   c. swimming pool chemicals.
   d. prescription drugs.

9. Injuries that result when ligaments and others tissues around a joint are stretched or torn are called
   a. fractures.
   b. strains.
   c. sprains.
   d. ruptures.

10. A head injury can result from a(n)
    a. auto accident.
    b. fall.
    c. assault.
    d. All of the above

11. A significant factors in many drowning cases is
   a. alcohol.
   b. exhaustion.
   c. sun exposure.
   d. hypothermia.

12. Victims of heatstroke may have all of the following symptoms, *except*
   a. hot, dry, flushed skin.
   b. disorientation.
   c. high body temperature.
   d. low blood pressure.

13. The heat related injury that results from excessive loss of salt and water is
   a. hyperthermia.
   b. heat exhaustion.
   c. heat stroke.
   d. hyperexhaustion.

14. What is the most painful heat-related injury?
   a. hyperthermia
   b. heat stroke
   c. heat cramps
   d. heat exhaustion

15. If you provide first aid to a victim of hypothermia, you should do all of the following, except
   a. make sure the person is evenly warmed using blankets, heating pads or hot water bottles.
   b. give the victim alcohol or caffeinated beverages to warm them.
   c. replace wet clothing.
   d. do not allow the victim to exercise.

Practice Test #2

1. The risk of dying in an auto crash is highest among
   a. drivers 16-24 years of age.
   b. drivers 25-34 years of age.
   c. drivers 45-54 years of age.
   d. drivers 55 years of age and older.

2. When someone stops breathing, you should
   a. perform mouth-to-mouth resuscitation.
   b. begin cardiopulmonary resuscitation.
   c. proceed with the Heimlich maneuver.
   d. apply pressure to the abdominal area.

3. The number of breaths given in rescue breathing to a child is to
   a. two breaths every three seconds.
   b. two breaths every five seconds.
   c. one breath every four seconds.
   d. one breath every ten seconds.

4. What is the universal sign of distress related to choking?
   a. pain in the left arm
   b. clasping of the throat with one or both hands
   c. being unable to talk
   d. clutching the chest over the heart

5. The method to control external bleeding that involves applying firm pressure by covering the wound with sterile dressing, bandage, or clean cloth is called
   a. direct pressure.
   b. indirect pressure.
   c. use of pressure points.
   d. elevation.

6. For minor burns caused by fire or scalding water, the best treatment is to
   a. apply running water or cold compresses for 20-30 minutes.
   b. put butter or grease on the burn.
   c. apply typical burn ointments to the burned areas.
   d. apply aloe vera to the burn.

7. A condition in which the cardiovascular system fails to provide sufficient blood circulation to all parts of the body is called
   a. heart attack.
   b. stroke.
   c. shock.
   d. cardiovascular obstruction.

8. When your car breaks down, you should
   a. try to get off the road as far as possible.
   b. set out flares or reflective triangles.
   c. stay in your car until a law enforcement officer arrives.
   d. All of the above

9. A break in the bone, including chips, cracks, splinters, and complete breaks, are called
   a. fractures.
   b. sprains.
   c. strains.
   d. compound breaks.

10. All head injuries can potentially lead to
   a. brain damage.
   b. cessation of breathing.
   c. cessation of pulse.
   d. All of the above

11. For severe head injuries, it is important to
   a. check the airway for breathing.
   b. check for fluid flowing from the ears or nose.
   c. remove any objects imbedded in the person's skull.
   d. Both a and b.

12. A condition of generalized cooling of the body resulting from exposure to cold temperatures or immersion in cold water is called
   a. hyperthermia.
   b. hypothermia.
   c. frostbite.
   d. shock.

13. Alcohol overdose is considered a medical emegency when
   a. a person has an irregular heartbeat.
   b. a person is in a coma.
   c. a person has warm, moist skin.
   d. Either a or b

14. To treat a victim of heat exhaustion, you should
   a. get the victim out of the sun.
   b. have the victim lie down flat with their feet elevated.
   c. replace lost fluids slowly and steadily.
   d. All of the above

15. To relieve the symptoms of heat cramps, the victim should
   a. be immersed in cool water.
   b. drink electrolyte-rich beverages.
   c. be placed by a fan.
   d. drink alcohol or caffeinated beverages.

Answers

CHAPTER 1

Answers to General Review Questions

1. Physical, Social, Mental, Emotional, Environmental, and Spiritual Health.
2. Prevention is taking positive actions now to avoid even becoming sick; primary, secondary, and tertiary prevention
3. Predisposing, enabling, and reinforcing factors.
4. Perceived seriousness of the health problem; perceived susceptibility to the health problem; cues to action.
5. Frequency, duration, seriousness, basis for problem behavior, antecedents.

Answers to Practice Test #1

1. C	6. D	11. D
2. D	7. D	12. A
3. A	8. A	13. B
4. B	9. C	14. D
5. B	10. A	15. A

Answers to Practice Test #2

1. A	6. B	11. A
2. A	7. B	12. B
3. A	8. C	13. D
4. C	9. C	14. A
5. D	10. D	15. D

CHAPTER 2

Answers to General Review Questions

1. They feel good about themselves, feel comfortable with other people, control tension and anxiety, able to meet the demands of life, curb hate and guilt, maintain a positive outlook, enrich the lives of others, cherish the things that make them smile, value diversity, and appreciate nature.
2. Psychoanalysis, psychodynamic, humanistic and Gestalt, behavior and cognitive-behavior, family and couples therapy.
3. Hereditary traits, hormonal functioning, physical health status, physical fitness level, and selected elements of mental and emotional health.
4. Family history of suicide, previous suicide attempts, excessive drug and alcohol use, prolonged depression, financial difficulties, serious illness in contemplator or loved ones.
5. Find a support group, complete required tasks, form realistic expectations, take/make time for self, maintain physical health, examine problems and seek help.

Answers to Practice Test #1

1. A	6. C	11. B
2. C	7. B	12. B
3. D	8. C	13. B
4. A	9. D	14. A
5. A	10. B	15. B

Answers to Practice Test #2

1. B	6. B	11. A
2. C	7. D	12. C
3. A	8. A	13. D
4. B	9. A	14. C
5. B	10. B	15. A

CHAPTER 3

Answers to General Review Questions

1. Alarm, Resistance, and Exhaustion.
2. Psychosocial factors such as changes, hassles, pressure, inconsistent goals and objectives, conflict, overload and burnout, environmental stressors (i.e., natural and man-made disasters), and self-imposed stress.

3. Type A personalities are hard-driving, competitive, anxious, time-driven, impatient, angry, and perfectionistic. Type B personalities are relaxed and noncompetitive.
4. Control, commitment, and challenge.
5. Increases the predictability of stressful events, fosters coping skills, generates self-talking, encourages confidence about successful outcomes, builds a commitment to personal action and responsibility for an adaptive course of action.

Answers to Practice Test #1

1. C	6. C	11. A
2. B	7. A	12. A
3. C	8. C	13. A
4. C	9. B	14. A
5. A	10. D	15. A

Answers to Practice Test #2

1. A	6. A	11. A
2. D	7. B	12. A
3. B	8. B	13. D
4. D	9. D	14. B
5. C	10. C	15. C

CHAPTER 4

Answers to General Review Questions

1. Tension building, Acute battering, Remorse/ reconciliation.
2. Poverty, unemployment, hopelessness, lack of education, inadequate housing, poor parental role models, cultural beliefs that objectify women and empower men to act as aggressors, lack of social support systems, discrimination, ignorance about people who are different, religious self-righteousness, breakdowns in the criminal justice system, stress and economic uncertainty.
3. Minimization, trivialization, blaming the victim, and "boys will be boys."
4. Gangs provide sense of belonging to a "family" and economic security.
5. Ask harasser to stop, document harassment, complain to a higher. (Remember that you have not done anything wrong.)

Answers to Practice Test #1

1. C	6. D	11. B
2. A	7. D	12. C
3. B	8. C	13. A
4. D	9. D	14. C
5. C	10. D	15. C

Answers to Practice Test #2

1. D	6. A	11. A
2. C	7. D	12. C
3. C	8. C	13. C
4. B	9. B	14. B
5. D	10. D	15. B

CHAPTER 5

Answers to General Review Questions

1. Approval and a sense of purpose in life, intimacy, social integration, nurturant; assistance reassurance or affirmation of our own worth.
2. All the characteristics of friendship (enjoyment, acceptance, trust, respect, mutual assistance, confiding, understanding, spontaneity) as well as fascination, exclusiveness, sexual desire, giving the utmost, being a champion, advocate.
3. Inhibited psychological growth rather than encouraging self-love, emotional expression, and individual growth.
4. Overdependence on the relationship, high value on sexual exclusivity, severity of the threat, low self-esteem, and fear of losing control.
5. While the reasons are numerous, such reasons include: tragedies such as the death of a child, serious illness of one's partner, severe financial reverses, career failure, breakdown in communication and cooperation between partners, unmet expectations regarding marriage itself or personal roles within the marriage.

Answers to Practice Test #1

1. C	6. A	11. D
2. D	7. A	12. B
3. B	8. A	13. B
4. A	9. B	14. D
5. D	10. D	15. B

Answers to Practice Test #2

1. D	6. D	11. A
2. D	7. B	12. B
3. D	8. A	13. A
4. C	9. D	14. C
5. C	10. C	15. B

CHAPTER 6

Answers to General Review Questions

1. Females: breast development, enlargement of external genitalia, growth of pubic hair, deposits of fat on hips and buttocks, and fine-textured skin and body hair. Males: growth of facial and body hair, deepening of voice, broadening of shoulders, and harrowing of hips.
2. Excitement/arousal, plateau, orgasm, and resolution. In males: refractory.
3. Gender roles are defined as the expression of maleness or femaleness exhibited on a daily basis.
4. Any behavior is normal which (1) you both enjoy, (2) hurts nobody, (3) is not associated with anxiety, (4) does not cut down your scope.
5. Sexual desire disorders, sexual arousal disorders, orgasm disorders, and sexual pain disorders.

Answers to Practice Test #1

1. B	6. B	11. A
2. C	7. D	12. A
3. A	8. C	13. B
4. C	9. D	14. B
5. C	10. C	15. B

Answers to Practice Test #2

1. B	6. A	11. B
2. C	7. B	12. B
3. D	8. D	13. A
4. A	9. B	14. D
5. D	10. B	15. C

CHAPTER 7

Answers to General Review Questions

1. A viable egg, a viable sperm, and possible access to the egg by the sperm.
2. For early detection of fetal abnormalities and the identification of high-risk mothers and infants.
3. Missed period, breast tenderness, extreme fatigue, sleeplessness, emotional upset, nausea, and vomiting.
4. Suppresses ovulation, prevents growth of uterine lining, and thickens the cervical mucus.
5. Infection, incomplete abortion, excessive bleeding, and cervical and uterine trauma. Also, in second trimester abortions: increased risk of uterine perforation, bleeding, infection, and incomplete abortion because the uterine wall becomes thinner as the pregnancy progresses.

Answers to Practice Test #1

1. A	6. A	11. D
2. B	7. B	12. B
3. D	8. C	13. B
4. C	9. D	14. B
5. B	10. C	15. B

Answers to Practice Test #2

1. A	6. B	11. B
2. C	7. C	12. C
3. B	8. A	13. D
4. C	9. B	14. A
5. A	10. A	15. D

CHAPTER 8

Answers to General Review Questions

1. Personal preferences, habit, ethnic heritage or tradition, social interactions, availability, emotional comfort, values, body image, and nutrition.
2. Proteins (12% of total calories), carbohydrates (48% of total calories from complex carbohydrates; 10% of total calories from simple carbohydrates), fats (no more than 30% of total calories), water, vitamins, minerals.
3. Vegans: avoid all food of animal origin; lacto-vegetarians: avoid flesh foods but eat dairy products; ovo-vegetarians: avoid flesh foods but eat eggs; lacto-ovo-vegetarians: avoid flesh foods but eat both dairy products and eggs; pesco-vegetarians: avoid meat but eat fish, diary products, and eggs; semivegetarians eat chicken, fish, dairy products, and eggs.
4. Depending on the contaminant eaten, symptoms vary tremendously. Symptoms may appear as early as a half hour after eating or they may take several days or weeks to develop. In most people, they come on 5-8 hours after eating and last only a day or two.
5. Buy fruits and vegetables in season; use coupons and specials; shop at discount warehouse food chains; plan ahead to avoid extra trips to store; purchase meats and other products in volume; cook large meals and freeze smaller portions; drain off fat.

Answers to Practice Test #1

1. D	6. A	11. B
2. B	7. D	12. B
3. B	8. D	13. C
4. B	9. C	14. B
5. D	10. A	15. B

Answers to Practice Test #2

1. C	6. C	11. B
2. D	7. C	12. A
3. B	8. A	13. C
4. D	9. D	14. B
5. D	10. C	15. B

CHAPTER 9

Answers to General Review Questions

1. Television, movies, magazines, beautiful models, athletic male superstars, warnings of the dangers of obesity from legitimate health organizations.
2. Social physique anxiety is a problem seen in both young men and women, in which the desire to look good has a destructive effect on a person's ability to function effectively socially.
3. The thyroid gland produces a hormone that regulates metabolism. While many people feel that an underactive thyroid impeded their ability to burn calories, most authorities agree that only 3-5% of the obese population have a thyroid problem.
4. The amount of muscle mass moved, the amount of weight being moved, and the amount of time the activity takes.
5. Anorexia nervosa, bulimia nervosa, and binge eating disorder.

Answers to Practice Test #1

1. B	6. B	11. B
2. A	7. C	12. C
3. B	8. C	13. A
4. A	9. B	14. D
5. B	10. B	15. B

Answers to Practice Test #2

1. C	6. C	11. C
2. A	7. B	12. B
3. C	8. A	13. A
4. C	9. B	14. B
5. B	10. B	15. B

CHAPTER 10

Answers to General Review Questions

1. Physical activity is any force exerted by skeletal muscles that results in energy usage above the level used when the body's systems are at rest.
2. Cardiorespiratory endurance, flexibility, muscular strength and endurance, body composition.
3. Calculated as the percentage of maximum heart rate (220) minus age; heart rate (pulse) taken during aerobic exercise to check of exercise intensity is at the desired level (i.e., 70 percent of maximum heart rate).
4. Flexibility enhances your efficiency of movement and your posture; flexibility exercises reduce the incidence and severity of musculo-tendinous injuries; and stretching exercises can enhance psychological as well as physical well-being.
5. RICE: Rest, ice, compression, and elevation.

Answers to Practice Test #1

1. A	6. D	11. D
2. D	7. C	12. A
3. C	8. D	13. B
4. D	9. A	14. B
5. D	10. C	15. B

Answers to Practice Test #2

1. B	6. D	11. C
2. C	7. B	12. C
3. C	8. C	13. C
4. B	9. B	14. A
5. C	10. D	15. B

CHAPTER 11

Answers to General Review Questions

1. (1) The presence of an abstinence syndrome--withdrawal; (2) an association pattern of pathological behavior; (3) relapse.
2. Compulsion characterized by obsession; loss of control; negative consequences; and denial.
3. Emotional pain; craving for relief; preoccupation with substance/behavior; substance use or compulsive behavior; short term pain relief; negative consequences resulting from behavior; depression or guilt or shame; more pain, low self-esteem.
4. Emphasizing care and concern for the addicted person; describing the behavior; expressing how the behavior affects the addict; outlining specifically what should be done.
5. Biopsychosocial model of addiction.

Answers to Practice Test #1

1. D	6. A	11. D
2. B	7. D	12.C
3. B	8. C	13. B
4. A	9. A	14. C
5. B	10. A	15. B

Answers to Practice Test #2

1. B	6. C	11. D
2.D	7. D	12. B
3. A	8. B	13. A
4. B	9. A	14. C
5. D	10. B	15. D

CHAPTER 12

Answers to General Review Questions

1. The alcohol concentration in the drink, the amount of alcohol consumed, the amount of food in the stomach, pylorospasm, and the person's mood.

2. Impairs the body's ability to recognize and fight foreign bodies such as bacteria and viruses.
3. An inability to develop social attachments, a need to be in control of all emotions and situations, low self-esteem, and depression.
4. $185 billion
5. When they have a turning point or dramatic occurrence: a spouse walks out, taking children and possessions; the boss issues an ultimatum; a courtroom judge offers the alternatives or prison or a treatment; when confronted by a friend or colleague.

Answers to Practice Test #1

1. C	6. C	11. C
2. D	7. D	12. D
3. A	8. B	13. C
4. B	9. A	14. A
5. A	10. A	15. A

Answers to Practice Test #2

1. A	6. D	11. A
2. C	7. D	12. C
3. C	8. D	13. B
4. B	9. D	14. C
5. A	10. D	15. C

CHAPTER 13

Answers to General Review Questions

1. Particulate matter, tar, benzopyrene, phenol, carbon monoxide, hydrogen cyanide, and hydrocarbons.
2. Increased heart and respiratory rate, constriction of blood vessels, increased blood pressure, decreased stomach contractions, decreased blood sugar levels, decreased sensation of the taste buds, reduction in appetite.
3. Color changes or lumps inside the lips; white, smooth or scaly patches in the mouth or on the neck, lips, or tongue; a red spot or sore on the lips or gums or inside the mouth that does not heal in two weeks; repeatedly bleeding in the mouth, difficulty or abnormality in speaking or swallowing.
4. Aversion therapy (pairs the act of smoking with some sort of noxious stimulus so that smoking itself is perceived as unpleasant); operant strategies (Pairs the act of smoking with an external stimulus); Self-control (identifies specific situations and teaching smokers the skills necessary to resist smoking).
5. It does not appear to be linked to high blood pressure, strokes, or heart disease. However, people who suffer from irregular heartbeat should be cautions. Coffee can contribute to ulcers and has been linked with fibrocystic breast cancer.

Answers to Practice Test #1

1. C	6. B	11. A
2. C	7. A	12. D
3. D	8. A	13. C
4. B	9. D	14. A
5. D	10. C	15. D

Answers to Practice Test #2

1. A	6. C	11. D
2. A	7. C	12. B
3. D	8. B	13. D
4. D	9. B	14. A
5. A	10. C	15. D

CHAPTER 14

Answers to General Review Questions

1. Prescription drugs, over-the-counter drugs, recreational drugs, herbal preparations, illicit dugs, and commercial preparations.

2. Brain damage, heart defects, kidney problems, and malformed heads, arms and fingers. They seem to be unable to respond or relate to people the way normal babies do, they are difficult to console and comfort. They have a significant increase in the risk of crib death.

3. Slightly increased heart rate, elevated blood pressure and temperature, goose flesh, increased reflex speeds, muscle tremors and twitches, perspiration, increased salivation, chills, headaches, and mild nausea. Can cause uterine muscle contractions and lead to premature labor and miscarriage in pregnant women.
4. Young men to increase their strength, power, bulk, and speed.
5. Multimodal approach.

Answers to Practice Test #1

1. B	6. B	11. D
2. A	7. B	12. D
3. C	8. D	13. B
4. C	9. B	14. B
5. A	10. C	15. B

Answers to Practice Test #2

1. B	6. A	11. A
2. B	7. A	12. B
3. D	8. A	13. A
4. D	9. B	14. B
5. A	10. B	15. D

CHAPTER 15

Answers to General Review Questions

1. Heredity, age, obesity, smoking, exercise, cholesterol levels, gender, systolic and diastolic blood pressure, stress, present heart disease symptoms, past personal history, diabetes.
2. Heredity, age, gender, and race.
3. Rest, drugs that affect: 1) the blood supply to the heart muscle and 2) the heart's demand for oxygen.
4. Kidney disease, obesity, or tumors of the adrenal glands.
5. Physicians may often be gender-biased in their delivery of health care, physicians tend to view male heart disease as a more severe problem, and women decline major procedures more often than men do.

Answers to Practice Test #1

1. C	6. B	11. A
2. C	7. C	12. C
3. D	8. D	13. B
4. C	9. C	14. B
5. A	10. D	15. D

Answers to Practice Test #2

1. C	6. A	11. B
2. B	7. C	12. C
3. A	8. A	13. C
4. C	9. B	14. B
5. A	10. A	15. D

CHAPTER 16

Answers to General Review Questions

1. Carcinomas, sarcomas, lymphomas, and leukemia.
2. Persistent cough, blood streaked sputum, chest pain, and recurrent attacks of pneumonia or bronchitis.
3. A: Asymmetry, half of the mole does not match the other half; B: Border irregularity, the edges are ragged, notched, or blurred; C: Color, pigmentation is not uniform; D: Diameter greater than six millimeters.
4. Magnetic resonance imagery uses magnetic fields, radio waves, and computers; computerized axial tomography uses radiation to view internal organs not normally visible by x-rays.

5. Stop smoking; avoid excessive sunlight; avoid excessive alcohol consumption, do not use smokeless tobacco; properly monitor estrogen use; avoid excessive radiation exposure; avoid occupational exposures to carcinogens; control your diet.

Answers to Practice Test #1

1. C	6. C	11. D
2. D	7. B	12. A
3. D	8. D	13. A
4. A	9. B	14. A
5. B	10. D	15. A

Answers to Practice Test #2

1. B	6. C	11. C
2. D	7. B	12. C
3. B	8. A	13. C
4. A	9. C	14. A
5. B	10. B	15. B

CHAPTER 17

Answers to General Review Questions

1. Susceptible host, disease agent, and environment. In addition, heredity, age, environmental conditions, and lifestyle.
2. Direct contact, indirect contact, food-borne infection, animal-borne infection, and water-borne infection.
3. Bacteria - Toxic shock syndrome, strep throat, tuberculosis; Viruses - common cold, influenza, hepatitis; Rickettsia - Rocky Mountain spotted fever, typhus; Fungi - Candidiasis, athlete's foot, ringworm; Protozoa - Trichomoniasis, giardiasis; Parasitic Worms - tapeworms, pinworms.
4. Skin; mucous membranes in the respiratory track and other linings of the body; cilia; tears, nasal secretions, ear wax, and other secretions found at the body's entrances.
5. Women.

Answers to Practice Test #1

1. C	6. D	11. B
2. C	7. B	12. C
3. B	8. D	13. B
4. A	9. B	14. C
5. A	10. A	15. C

Answers to Practice Test #2

1. B	6. B	11. A
2. C	7. A	12. C
3. D	8. D	13. B
4. A	9. A	14. A
5. D	10. B	15. B

CHAPTER 18

Answers to General Review Questions

1. Molds, animal dander (hair and dead skin), pollen, ragweed, or dust.
2. Female, fat, fair, forty, and flatulent.
3. Between ages 20 and 45; women lifting heavy objects quickly; very tall and overweight or lanky body types; poor posture; lower overall trunk strength and total level of fitness and conditioning; psychological factors including depression, apathy, inattentiveness, boredom, emotional upsets, drug abuse, and family and financial problems; occupations such as truck drivers and materials handlers; smokers or persons with chronic coughs.
4. Major criteria: debilitating fatigue that persists for at least six months, ad the absence of diagnosis of other illnesses that could cause the symptoms; minor criteria: headaches, fever, sore throat, painful lymph nodes, weakness, fatigue after exercise, sleep problems, and rapid onset of these symptoms.
5. Injuries to nerves, soft tissue, or joints that result from the physical stress of repeated motions.

Answers to Practice Test #1

1. C	6. C	11. C
2. A	7. C	12. A
3. A	8. C	13. C
4. B	9. C	14. B
5. D	10. A	15. D

Answers to Practice Test #2

1. B	6. B	11. A
2. D	7. B	12. C
3. B	8. B	13. D
4. A	9. B	14. A
5. A	10. B	15. D

CHAPTER 19

Answers to General Review Questions

1. Erik Erikson and Robert Peck emphasized adaptation and adjustment as related to self-development. Erikson stated that people must progress through eight critical stages during their life-times. Peck focuses on the critical issues of middle and old age. Key to both theories is the age-related factors of lifelong behavior patterns.
2. Today, the elderly require approximately 38% of total national health care costs, with estimated costs in excess of $6,800.
3. Gender, age, low bone mass, early menopause, thin, small-framed body, race, lack of calcium, lack of physical activity, cigarette smoking, alcohol and/or caffeine abuse, and heredity.
4. Given an appropriate length of time, elderly people may learn and develop skills in a similar manner to younger people. What elderly people may lack in speed of learning, they make up for in practical knowledge.
5. People who have aged successfully have the following characteristics: they have managed to avoid debilitating diseases and disability; they are able to maintain a level of physical functioning, live independently and engage in most normal activities of daily living; they have maintained their cognitive functioning; they have sustained an active engagement in social and productive activities; and they are resilient.

Answers to Practice Test #1

1. B	6. D	11. A
2. A	7. A	12. D
3. A	8. A	13. D
4. A	9. B	14. C
5. B	10. B	15. A

Answers to Practice Test #2

1. A	6. C	11. D
2. D	7. A	12. B
3. A	8. A	13. A
4. C	9. B	14. A
5. D	10. B	15. D

CHAPTER 20

Answers to General Review Questions

1. Irreversible cessation of circulatory and respiratory functions, or irreversible cessation of all functions of the entire brain, including the brainstem.
2. Modern technology, personal experiences, the environment, age, problems with access to health care, and many other factors can influence our attitudes about death and dying.
3. Denial, anger, bargaining, depression, and acceptance.

4. Those who argue in favor of PAS offer the following arguments: respect for autonomy, justice, compassion, individual liberty versus state interest, and openness of discussion. Those who argue against PAS offer arguments such as: sanctity of life, passive versus active distinction, potential for abuse, professional integrity, and fallibility of the profession.
5. Electrical or mechanical resuscitation of the heart, mechanical respiration by machine, nasogastric tube feedings, intravenous nutrition, gastrostomy, medications to treat life-threatening infections.

Answers to Practice Test #1

1. C	6. D	11. C
2. A	7. C	12. C
3. C	8. C	13. A
4. D	9. C	14. C
5. B	10. B	15. B

Answers to Practice Test #2

1. B	6. B	11. A
2. B	7. C	12. C
3. C	8. C	13. A
4. A	9. C	14. C
5. D	10. D	15. C

CHAPTER 21

Answers to General Review Questions

1. Environmental degradation caused by loss of top soil, pesticides, toxic residues, deforestation, global warming, air pollution, and acid rain.
2. Woodstoves, furnaces, asbestos, passive smoke, formaldehyde, and radon.
3. A rapid rise in the production of greenhouse gases. Trees transform carbon dioxide into oxygen.
4. Soil erosion and sedimentation, construction wastes, pesticide and fertilizer runoff, urban street runoff, wastes from engineering projects, acid mine drainage, leakage from septic tanks, and sewage sludge.
5. Recycle, reuse, and reduce the products we use.

Answers to Practice Test #1

1. D	6. A	11. B
2. A	7. A	12. B
3. C	8. D	13. D
4. A	9. D	14. A
5. B	10. D	15. D

Answers to Practice Test #2

1. C	6. B	11. B
2. A	7. C	12. B
3. A	8. A	13. B
4. C	9. D	14. D
5. C	10. A	15. D

CHAPTER 22

Answers to General Review Questions

1. Nonprofit hospitals generally reinvest their earnings in the hospital for improving health care and often care for patients whether they could pay or not. Proprietary hospitals do not receive tax breaks and provide far less charity care.
2. Surgicenters, freestanding emergency centers, urgicenters, freestanding imaging and diagnostic laboratory centers, trauma centers, and health clinics.
3. Cost, access, malpractice, unnecessary procedures, complicated and cumbersome insurance, and dramatic ranges in quality.
4. For a drug to be switched from prescription to OTC status, it must meet the following criteria: the drug has been marketed as a prescription drug for at least three years; the use of the drug has been relatively high during the time it was available as a prescription drug; adverse drug reactions not alarming, and the frequency of side effects has not increased during the time the drug was available to the public.
5. The staff model, the group network model, and the independent practice association.

Answers to Practice Test #1

1. C	6. C	11. B
2. C	7. A	12. D
3. A	8. A	13. D
4. B	9. C	14. A
5. D	10. D	15. B

Answers to Practice Test #2

1. B	6. B	11. B
2. C	7. D	12. B
3. A	8. A	13. B
4. B	9. C	14. B
5. C	10. B	15. B

CHAPTER 23

Answers to General Review Questions

1. Chiropractic treatment, acupuncture, herbalists and homeopaths, and naturopathy.
2. Antioxidants are quite popular, with the primary antioxidants being betacarotene, selenium, vitamin C, and vitamin E.
3. Yoga, tai chi, and body work.
4. The German Commission E attempts to regulate the sale of alternative medicines and supplements.
5. Those who seek CAM tend to be more educated, middle-aged, and have a middle-class socioeconomic status.

Answers to Practice Test #1

1. C	6. C	11. D
2. C	7. C	12. B
3. A	8. B	13. B
4. D	9. D	14. A
5. C	10. B	15. A

Answers to Practice Test #2

1. A	6. B	11. D
2. A	7. D	12. C
3. A	8. B	13. C
4. B	9. A	14. D
5. C	10. D	15. B

APPENDIX A

Answers to General Review Questions

1. Laws that grant immunity (protection from civil liability if you act in good faith to provide care to the best of your ability, according to your level of training).
2. Symptoms of shock; coughing up or vomiting blood; blood in urine; black, tarlike stools; and, abdominal discomfort or pain (rigidity or spasms).
3. Children under the age of 5.
4. Temperatures below 32 degrees F.
5. Shivering; vague, slow, slurred speech; poor judgment; lethargy, or extreme exhaustion; slowed breathing and heartbeat; and, numbness and loss of feeling in extremities.

Answers to Practice Test #1

1. D	6. D	11. A
2. C	7. B	12. D
3. D	8. A	13. B
4. C	9. C	14. C
5. B	10. D	15. B

Answers to Practice Test #2

1. A	6. A	11. D
2. A	7. C	12. B
3. C	8. D	13. D
4. B	9. A	14. D
5. A	10. D	15. B